AN INVITATION TO HEALTH
Fourth Edition

Test Bank

Christopher Cooke, M.S.
Division of Community Health Service
School of Public Health
University of North Carolina at Chapel Hill
Chapel Hill, North Carolina

Acknowledgements
Special thanks to Mary Bobbitt-Cooke, Health Promotion Program Coordinator,
Orange County Health Department, Hillsborough, North Carolina.

ISBN 0-8053-0155-0

ABCDEFGHIJ-AL-8932109

The Benjamin/Cummings Publishing Company
390 Bridge Parkway
Redwood City, California 94065

AN INVITATION TO HEALTH
Test Bank

Preface

The test bank to the fourth edition of <u>An Invitation to Health</u> reflects the text's increased emphasis on the importance of "health directed behavior." Health educators who work directly with clients interested in health promotion and disease prevention, as well as scholars in the field of health, readily acknowledge that just learning about the health consequences of behavior rarely sustains the motivation necessary to make lasting changes. While the primary function of this text is to educate the student about health, its stress on the importance of integrating knowledge into daily life is to be commended.

In order to respond to the health activation information in the text, and still provide comprehensive content coverage of the academic material, the test bank makes use of a variety of types of questions.

<u>True-False</u> True-false questions are used to test the student's knowledge of basic concepts, facts, and definitions. The global nature of the information tested in these questions provides a critical context for more detailed or applied knowledge. Mastery of information at this level is necessary in order for the student to appreciate the relevance of more detailed material.

<u>Multiple Choice</u> Multiple choice questions test the student's ability to distinguish or manipulate sets of information that relate to a single concept. While the structure of this type of test item makes correct guessing more difficult than true-false questions, it still requires the student to identify or choose the correct answer rather than provide it from what he or she has learned.

<u>Completion</u> The completion questions require the student to recall sets of information critical to the application of knowledge. These questions are drawn primarily from the "Strategy for Change" sections of the text, and mastery of these items indicates the student's capacity to make directed behavior change if he or she desires to do so.

<u>Matching</u> Many chapters in the text introduce systems of information that require detailed knowledge of definitions, titles, and functions. Note that each matching question has at least one additional choice in the answer column to prevent matching by deduction.

<u>Essay</u> Essay questions offer the student an opportunity to demonstrate their ability to apply knowledge to the world around them. They also allow the instructor a chance to communicate a particular emphasis to the material in the text by selecting among the issues covered in these questions.

Test bank items may be used individually or in groups, and have been laid out in order to facilitate ease of duplication and separation of questions from answers. Topic and page references are also provided. It is my hope that this test bank will not only provide a reliable assessment of learned knowledge, but will also help to underscore the importance of application and health directed behavior.

Christopher Cooke
Chapel Hill, North Carolina
October, 1988

TABLE OF CONTENTS

<u>**AN INVITATION TO HEALTH**</u>
TEST BANK

Section I - Your Mind: The Quest for Understanding

<u>Chapter 1: An Invitation to Health</u>

In this chapter -

* Health and Wellness
* Mind-Body-Spirit
* Taking Responsibility

Section I - Your Mind: The Quest for Understanding
Chapter 1: An Invitation to Health

True-False

1/1   False
       Health/Wellness
       Page #3

The World Health Organization (WHO) defines health as "the absence of disease or infirmity."

1/2   True
       Health/Wellness
       Page #3

The term holistic health refers to an approach to health that emphasizes the complete person - physical, mental, and spiritual.

1/3   True
       Health/Wellness
       Page #4

Most fatal illnesses today are the result of personal lifestyle choices.

1/4   False
       Mind-Body-Spirit
       Page #4

The relationship between spiritual fulfillment and personal well-being is not considered significant by Americans involved in the wellness movement.

1/5   True
       Taking Responsibility
       Page #5

Data from a national survey show that the number of adults who exercise regularly now exceeds two-thirds of the population.

1/6   True
       Taking Responsibility
       Page #5

According to a recent Gallup poll, individuals with the greatest sense of control over their health feel happier and more satisfied with life.

1/7   False
       Taking Responsibility
       Page #6

Values and beliefs do not significantly affect your ability to change unhealthy habits.

1/8   True
       Taking Responsibility
       Page #6

The individual process of changing from a bad or unhealthy habit to a healthy one involves a series of common and predictable "stages".

1/9   True
       Taking Responsibility
       Page #7

Preventive care and wellness programs have actually reduced the incidence of death and illness caused by cardio-vascular disease, cancer, and auto-mobile accidents.

Chapter 1: An Invitation to Health

1/10   False
        Taking Responsibility
        Page #9

The individual most responsible for your health is your personal physician.

Multiple Choice

1/11   b.
        Health/Wellness
        Page #3

The World Health Organization defines health as

a. the absence of disease or infirmity.
b. complete physical, mental, and social well-being.
c. responding promptly to early signs of health problems.
d. an ever-expanding experience of purposeful, enjoyable living.

1/12   d.
        Health/Wellness
        Page #3

Holistic health emphasizes self-responsibility in each of the following areas except one. Which is it?

a. preventive medical care
b. physical fitness
c. stress management
d. adequate health insurance

1/13   d.
        Health/Wellness
        Page #4

Which of the following is said to contribute to the state of wellness described as "an ever-expanding experience of purposeful, enjoyable living?"

a. avoiding conflict
b. believing in the sun even when it doesn't shine
c. working for justice and social change
d. trusting that your personal resources are your greatest strengths for living and growing

1/14   a.
        Health/Wellness
        Page #5

Of the ten leading causes of death in the U.S., half are related to

a. lifestyle choices.
b. environmental pollutants.
c. medical malpractice.
d. infectious diseases.

1/15   c.
Taking Responsibility
Page #5

Since 1970, the number of Americans involved in the movement toward wellness and fitness has

a. stayed about the same.
b. declined steadily.
c. increased steadily.
d. fluxuated up and down.

1/16   a.
Health/Wellness
Page #4

Which of the following measures is considered the most reliable indicator of a society's health?

a. infant mortality rate
b. life expectancy
c. overall fertility rate
d. live birth rate

1/17   d.
Health/Wellness
Page #4

Which of the following statements regarding the U.S. infant mortality rate is correct?

a. The rate reached its lowest level during the wellness movement of the 1970's.
b. The U.S. rate shows American society to be the healthiest in the world.
c. The rate has been rising steadily since AIDS was discovered.
d. The U.S. rate is high compared to other industrialized nations.

1/18   b.
Health/Wellness
Page #4

The primary cause of death before the age of 40 in the U.S. is

a. infectious diseases.
b. injuries caused by accidents, suicides, and violent crime.
c. chronic disease such as cancer and heart disease.
d. drug abuse.

1/19   c.
Health/Wellness
Page #4

Which of the following is not part of a strategy for achieving personal wellness?

a. communicating your feelings to other people
b. acting assertively
c. aggressively attacking problems that beset you
d. knowing your body's emotional and physical patterns or signals

3

1/20 d.
    Taking Responsibility
    Page #5

Health conscious Americans share one characteristic - they all

a. participate in some sort of exercise or diet program.
b. have given up unhealthy habits.
c. focus on one particular aspect of themselves.
d. take responsibility for improving their health and wellness.

1/21 b.
    Taking Responsibility
    Page #5

The three factors that have the most influence on behavior are predisposing, enabling, and

a. socializing
b. reinforcing
c. actualizing
d. affirming

1/22 c.
    Taking Responsibility
    Page #5

Predisposing factors that influence behavior include

a. skills, resources, and capacities that you will need to make positive changes in your behavior.
b. praise, rewards, encouragement, or recognition for meeting a goal.
c. knowledge, attitudes, beliefs, and values necessary to begin the process of behavior change.
d. hereditary traits, characteristics, or genetic qualities that affect your behavior.

1/23 a.
    Taking Responsibility
    Page #6

Researchers report that people are most likely to change health behavior if they believe that they (1) are at risk, (2) will suffer if they don't change, and (3) will

a. benefit from the change.
b. have access to assistance.
c. have friends and relatives to support them.
d. be able to change permanently.

1/24   b.
        Taking Responsibility
        Page #6

Efforts to successfully change health behavior depend, more than anything else, on

a. self-observation.
b. believing in success.
c. avoiding risky situations.
d. having a religious conversion.

1/25   c.
        Taking Responsibility
        Page #6

The first step toward changing a negative health behavior is

a. planning ahead to avoid temptation.
b. signing a contract for change.
c. awareness of risky behavior.
d. identifying cues for negative behavior.

1/26   d.
        Taking Responsibility
        Page #7

Which of the following is not part of a sound strategy for changing health behavior?

a. setting small, manageable goals
b. rewarding yourself regularly
c. expecting occasional relapses
d. focusing on long-term rewards

1/27   b.
        Taking Responsibility
        Page #7

What percentage of Americans don't know that cancer is usually caused by lifestyle choices? Choose the answer most nearly correct.

a. 40%
b. 50%
c. 60%
d. 70%

1/28   a.
        Taking Responsibility
        Page #7

A good strategy for helping another person change an unhealthy habit includes (1) saying how you feel about their behavior, (2) providing reasons for change, (3) offering rewards and encouragement, and

a. volunteering to help.
b. expecting complete success.
c. ignoring your own unhealthy behavior.
d. criticizing unsucccessful attempts at change.

1/29   d.
Taking Responsibility
Page #10

The entire process of maintaining or restoring health depends on

a. reliable information.
b. good medical care.
c. your environment.
d. decisions you make.

1/30   c.
Taking Responsibility
Page #8

An epidemiological study is one in which scientists

a. test a procedure in the laboratory.
b. use a double-blind technique.
c. assess the health status of a group.
d. test a theory using animals.

Essay

1/31   Identify the three types of factors that influence behavior, and describe how each of these factors might affect an individual's desire to make a specific behavior change (e.g., to stop smoking, or to lose weight).

1/32   Select a personal health behavior or habit you would like to change or improve. Design a plan for making your desired change that includes the following components:

- how you would develop and maintain awareness of the negative behavior
- what kind of situations would contribute to/detract from your desired change(s)
- how you would involve friends and/or family for support
- a set of short-term goals
- how you're going to deal with occasional relapses
- how you're going to reward yourself

1/33   Imagine that you have just finished reading a lengthy article on weight loss in a popular news magazine. The article made numerous recommendations about what approaches work best and are most reliable for long-term weight loss. Describe how you would evaluate the information in such an article. How would you go about gathering additional information, or validating what you've already read?

<u>AN INVITATION TO HEALTH</u>
TEST BANK

Section I - Your Mind: The Quest for Understanding

<u>Chapter 2: Emotional and Mental Health</u>

In this chapter -

* Psychological Health
* Personality Development
* Self-Understanding

AN INVITATION TO HEALTH
Test Bank

Section I - Your Mind: The Quest for Understanding
Chapter 2: Emotional and Mental Health

True-False

2/1	False Psychological Health Page #12	The term psychological health refers only to emotional states and feelings.
2/2	False Psychological Health Page #12	Psychological health refers to the absence of emotional problems or illness.
2/3	True Psychological Health Page #12	Mental health is the ability to form reasonable expectations based on accurate perceptions of reality.
2/4	False Personality Development Page #14	According to Piaget, personality development is determined by early childhood experiences.
2/5	True Personality Development Page #13	Sigmund Freud described the psyche as the "sum of all mental activity, both conscious and unconscious."
2/6	True Personality Development Page #14	The Swiss psychologist Piaget was concerned primarily with how we think, not what we think.
2/7	False Personality Development Page #15	Erikson maintained that the social environment had little impact on ego development.
2/8	False Personality Development Page #16	The humanist movement sees most people as basically the same at birth, with society directing individual development.
2/9	True Personality Development Page #19	Researchers have now identified developmental periods during adulthood.
2/10	True Self-Understanding Page #20	The valuing of oneself as a person is also known as self-esteem.
2/11	False Self-Understanding Page #23	Feelings have little, if any, effect on our physical health.

2/12   True
             Self-Understanding
             Page #26

The inappropriate use of defense mechanisms can lead to maladaptive behavior.

Multiple Choice

2/13   b
             Psychological Health
             Page #12

Emotional health can be defined as

a. the absence of emotional problems or illness.
b. the range of feelings and/or moods that people experience.
c. the ability to perceive reality.
d. being vigorous, happy, and self-confident.

2/14   a
             Psychological Health
             Page #12

Which of the following is not a requirement for psychological health

a. a high level of intelligence
b. the ability to love
c. a sense of self-worth
d. looking for work that matches one's skills and education

2/15   d
             Personality Development
             Page #13

Which one of the following people was responsible for the concept of the "psyche"?

a. Wordsworth
b. Rogers
c. Maslow
d. Freud

2/16   c
             Personality Development
             Page #13

Which of the following statements about Freud's theory is most accurate?

a. The psyche is the same as the ego.
b. The ego functions as a parent, separating right from wrong.
c. The id constantly seeks pleasure and gratification.
d. The superego is the primitive part of the unconscious.

2/17   a
             Personality Development
             Page #13

Freud called the psychic drive or energy associated with sexual instinct

a. the libido.
b. phallic phase.
c. the id.
d. the aggressive impulse.

2/18   b
        Personality Development
        Page #14

Who was responsible for describing personality development in stages of cognitive ability?

a. Erikson
b. Piaget
c. Kohlberg
d. Rogers

2/19   d
        Personality Development
        Pages #14-15

The sequence of stages of cognitive development include sensorimotor, preoperational, concrete, and

a. latent.
b. industrial.
c. dimensional.
d. formal.

2/20   c
        Personality Development
        Page #15

How many stages are there in Erikson's theory of ego development?

a. 3
b. 5
c. 8
d. 11

2/21   a
        Personality Development
        Page #15

Which of the following is _not_ one of the stages of ego development described by Erikson?

a. Convention versus Rebellion
b. Industry versus Inferiority
c. Autonomy versus Shame and Doubt
d. Generativity versus Self-absorption and Stagnation

2/22   c
        Personality Development
        Page #16

Which of the following statements about Mazlow's theory of self-actualization is most accurate?

a. A person is self-actualized if they have had a "peak experience."
b. Self-actualization is a more basic need than love or affection.
c. It is a state of wellness and fulfillment reached by satisfying needs.
d. People who are self-actualized tend to focus on themselves.

2/23   b
        Personality Development
        Page #19

Behavioral psychology attempts to explain behavior

a. by focusing on the ego's need for self-actualization.
b. without explaining what happens in the mind.
c. on the basis of how adults make choices.
d. by studying how children play.

2/24   d
        Personality Development
        Page #19

According to behavioral psychologists, individuals develop as a result of

a. genetic traits.
b. developmental crises.
c. positive stimulation.
d. conditioning.

2/25   b
        Self-Understanding
        Page #22

Your self-esteem is based primarily on

a. external factors such as wealth and appearance.
b. what you believe about yourself.
c. your ability to eliminate weaknesses from your personality.
d. the feedback you get from other people.

2/26   c
        Personality Development
        Page #19

Which of the following statements is most accurate regarding current research on adult development?

a. Men and women remain bound by sex roles throughout adult life.
b. Middle adult years are characterized by stagnation.
c. There is no single timetable that applies equally to men and women.
d. When you were born has little effect on how you experience life.

2/27   c
        Self-Understanding
        Page #24

Which of the following is the best definition of a value?

a. something you want to achieve
b. what you say you believe
c. what you use to judge people, events, and yourself
d. ideals that can never be reached

2/28   d
        Self-Understanding
        Page #26

Psychological devices for dealing with conflict and anxiety are called

a. REM sleep patterns.
b. affirmations.
c. hallucinations.
d. defense mechanisms.

2/29   b
        Self-Understanding
        Page #27

Which of the following statements about sleep is correct?

a. Each dream is full of hidden meanings.
b. Dream sleep periods are necessary for psychological well-being.
c. REM stands for Random Event Memory.
d. Gender has little effect on dream content and style.

2/30   b
        Self-Understanding
        Page #28

According to researchers at Stanford University, the percent of people who describe themselves as shy is

a. 20%
b. 40%
c. 60%
d. 80%

2/31   a
        Self-Understanding
        Page #27

Which of the following statements is an effective strategy for giving advice.

a. Don't be enthusiastic about just one suggestion.
b. Be judgemental.
c. Back up your advice with opinions.
d. Provide lots of information.

2/32   c
        Self-Understanding
        Page #29

Which of the following is a symptom of anxiety?

a. hallucinations
b. weariness
c. mental distraction
d. helplessness

2/33   b
        Self-Understanding
        Page #29

Clinical depression is marked by chronic hopelessness, despair, and

a. anxiety.
b. helplessness.
c. lowered blood pressure.
d. edginess.

2/34   d
        Self-Understanding
        Page #30

Which of the following statements about anger is most accurate?

a. The emotion of anger is usually absent during the first year of life.
b. Angry feelings are more likely to turn into aggression if they are expressed.
c. Aggressive people are most likely to have angry feelings.
d. The expression of anger can have positive results.

2/35   a
        Self-Understanding
        Page #30

Assertiveness is

a. the spontaneous recognition and expression of feelings.
b. forceful behavior used to control other people.
c. unrelated to the rights one has as an individual.
d. not an effective method for preventing the buildup of anger.

2/36   b
        Self-Understanding
        Page #31

Which of the following statements about sleep is _false_?

a. Sleep disturbance frequently has psychological causes.
b. Sleep patterns are unaffected by psychological states when awake.
c. About 30% of adults have trouble falling asleep, staying asleep, or staying awake during the day.
d. Sleep problems usually develop slowly.

Matching

2/37   Directions: Match each of the phases of Freud's theory of personality development on the left with its correct age period on the right. Each age period may be used only once.

	Phase		Age Period
1.	__ Oral	a.	school age
2.	__ Anal	b.	3 to 4 years old
3.	__ Phallic	c.	18 months to 3 years
4.	__ Oedipal	d.	puberty and adolescence
5.	__ Latency	d.	young adulthood
6.	__ Genital	e.	infancy to 18 months
		f.	over 65 years old
		g.	4-6 years old

1-f, 2-c, 3-b, 4-h, 5-a, 6-e
Personality Development
Page #13

2/38   Directions: Match each of the stages of Piaget's theory on the left with its correct description on the right. Each description may be used only once.

	Stage		Description
1.	__ Sensorimotor	a.	limited perspective and the ability to handle only small amounts of information
2.	__ Preoperational Thought	b.	becoming possessive of the oppposite-sex parent
3.	__ Concrete Operations	c.	abstract thinking and complex reasoning.
4.	__ Formal Operations	d.	seeking stimulation, exploring with the senses, developing mental images
		e.	developing confidence and a sense of mastery
		f.	dealing with several aspects of a problem, focusing on changes rather than states

1-d, 2-a, 3-f, 4-c
Personality Development
Pages #14-15

2/39   Directions: Match the developmental stage on the left with its
         corresponding developmental crisis on the right. Each crisis
         description may be used only once.

         <u>Stage</u>   <u>Crisis</u>

1. __ Trust vs Mistrust   a. inconsistent, impaired, or inade-
2. __ Autonomy vs Shame/Doubt   quate care from the mother
3. __ Initiative vs Guilt   b. inability to share love and develop
4. __ Industry vs Inferiority   close relationships
5. __ Ego Identity vs Role   c. failure to have developed beyond
       Confusion   self-absorption; memories of a life
6. __ Intimacy vs Isolation   without purpose
7. __ Generativity vs. Self-   d. failure to develop identity separate
       Absorption/Stagnation   from parents
8. __ Ego Integrity vs Despair   e. feeling ashamed or foolish, having
                                         doubts about judgement ability
                                      f. focusing on genitals as the source
                                         of sexual pleasure
                                      g. feeling badly about new behaviors,
                                         interests, or curiosity
                                      h. primary satisfaction comes from
                                         sucking, crying, and chewing
                                      i. inability to master challenges
                                      j. failure to pursue meaningful and
                                         socially useful tasks

         1-a, 2-e, 3-g, 4-i,
         5-d, 6-b, 7-j, 8-c
         Personality Development
         Pages #15-16

Completion

2/40   * id   What are the three aspects of the
         * ego   psyche as described by Freud?
         * superego   1. _____
         Personality Development   2. _____
         Page #13   3. _____

2/41   libido   Freud saw personality development as
         Personality Development   a process of psychosexual phases
         Page #13   fueled by psychic energy called the

                                      _____.

2/42   Ego Identify vs Role   James, a young man aged 28, still
            Confusion   lives at home and spends a great deal
         Personality Development   of time hanging around with old high
         Page #16   school friends. He consistently turns
                                      to his parents for assistance with
                                      difficult moral and ethical decisions.
                                      Which of Erikson's ego develoment
                                      stages most accurately characterizes
                                      James situation?

                                      _____

2/43   affirmation
        Self-Understanding
        Page #22

Janice is using a technique to build her self-esteem that involves repeating positive statements about her best personal qualities. What is this technique called?

_____

2/44   * Consider the consequen-
          ces of each choice
        * Choose freely from all
          alternatives
        * Publicly affirm your
          values
        * Act on your values
        Self-Understanding
        Page #24

Identify the four steps of values clarification.
1. _____
2. _____
3. _____
4. _____

2/45   resources
        Self-Understandiong
        Page #25

Dan decided to take a backpacking trip into the mountains. He bought a map, laid out a course, and then found out he didn't have enough money to buy the necessary equipment. He gave up and called off the trip. Before quitting, Dan should have gone on to the next step of problem solving and identified his _____.

2/46   projection
        Self-Understanding
        Page #26

Carla has been feeling discouraged about her relationship with Juan for some time, and wants to break up. When Juan decides to go bowling with friends instead of coming to visit, Carla is convinced that Juan is no longer interested in a relationship. What defense mechanism is most likely affecting Carla's thinking?

_____

2/47   assertiveness
        Self-Understanding
        Page #30

When you arrive at the service station to pick up your car, you notice that it's still out in the lot and hasn't been repaired. When you ask the service manager about it, she says you will have to wait several more days. You feel very angry, and decide to tell the service manager how you are feeling and what you want to happen. What is the name of this technique for being open and frank about your feelings and rights?

_____

Essay

2/48   Describe how emotional and mental health enable a person to "live to the fullest."

2/49   What are the critical differences in emphasis between Freud's, Erikson's, and Piaget's theories of personality development? Support your answer with examples.

2/50   Describe the role that feelings play in your daily life. How are concepts like self-esteem and self-concept linked to personal feelings?

<u>AN INVITATION TO HEALTH</u>
TEST BANK

Section I - Your Mind: The Quest for Understanding

<u>Chapter 3: Psychological Disorders</u>

In this chapter -

* Mental Illness
* Mood Disorders
* Anxiety Disorders
* Personality Disorders
* Eating Disorders
* Psychotherapy

Section I - Your Mind: The Quest for Understanding
Chapter 3: Psychological Disorders

True-False

3/1	False Mental Illness Page #35	A single standard of mental health is used to determine treatment for psychological disturbances.
3/2	False Mental Illness Page #35	Mental illness is directly related to personal strengths of the individual such as willpower and morality.
3/3	True Mental Illness Page #35	Karl Menninger's continuum represents a range of mental states based on the principle of organization.
3/4	True Mental Illness Page #36	The most severely disadvantaged group in terms of mental illness are American Indians.
3/5	False Mental Illness Page #36	Certain types of people are immune to psychological disorders.
3/7	True Mental Illness Page #37	Neurosis can be defined as any symptom that an individual finds unacceptable or distressing.
3/8	True Mood Disorders Page #38	Depression is the most common mood disorder.
3/9	True Mood Disorders Page #38	Depression can be characterized by an imbalance of important chemicals in the brain.
3/10	False Mood Disorders Page #43	Suicide is not a significant cause of death among young adults.
3/11	False Anxiety Disorders Page #45	Panic attacks are the most common anxiety disorders affecting Americans.
3/12	True Personality Disorders Page #46	Personal traits that impair a person's work or social life are called personality disorders.

3/13   False   Eating disorders affect men and women
           Eating Disorders   equally.
           Page #46

3/14   True   There is currently no cure for schizo-
           Schizophrenic Disorders phrenia.
           Page #51

3/15   True   Current research demonstrates that
           Psychotherapy   psychotherapy is effective for the
           Page #54   average person.

Multiple-Choice

3/16   c   Which of the following statements about
           Mental Illness   mental illness in America is most
           Page #36   accurate?

a. The majority of people with mental illness will never recover.
b. One out of every 25 adults will experience at least one episode of severe depression.
c. At any given time, one out of every five Americans is suffering from a psychological disorder requiring treatment.
d. Menninger viewed self-control and ego management as unrelated to good psychological adjustment.

3/17   a   Which of the following statements is
           Mental Illness   a myth about mental illness?
           Page #36

a. People with psychiatric problems are crazy all the time.
b. The majority of psychiatric disorders can be cured or controlled.
c. Even children are susceptible to psychological disorders.
d. No one is immune to psychological disorders.

3/18   d
         Mood Disorders
         Page #38

Which of the following statements about depression is most accurate?

a. The disease of depression is uncommon relative to other psychological disorders.
b. Of all the major psychiatric disorders, depression is one of the least studied and understood.
c. The rate of depression in young people has been falling recently.
d. The major components of depression include helplessness, despair, and hopelessness.

3/19   b
         Mood Disorders
         Pages #38-39

Which of the following sets of personal factors is the most accurate indicator of risk for depression?

a. poor physical health, married, white male, aged 35
b. female with family history of depression and recent personal trauma or illness
c. poor exercise and eating habits, female, unsatisfying "body image"
d. black male, recently divorced, in good physical health

3/20   c
         Mood Disorders
         Page #39

To meet the most recent criteria for a diagnosis of depression, patients must have continuous feelings of sadness, lack energy, have problems with thinking clearly, feel worthless, and

a. have a family history of depression.
b. experience hallucinations.
c. have lost interest or pleasure in activities.
d. have attempted suicide.

3/21   a
         Mood Disorders
         Pages #40-41

Which of the following statements about the treatment of depression is most accurate?

a. 90% of patients who get help improve within 3 to 6 weeks.
b. Without treatment, an episode of depression can last an average of 6 weeks.
c. According to the National Institute of Mental Health, drugs are more effective than talking therapies in the treatment of depression.
d. Seasonal Affective Disorder (SAD) is treated by sleep deprivation.

3/22   b
          Mood Disorders
          Page #43

Which of the following statements about suicide is <u>not</u> true?

a. Suicide is the second leading cause of death among those between the ages of 15 and 24.
b. Suicide is a mood disorder.
c. The suicide rate among college students, women in their twenties, and racial minorities has risen over the past 20 years.
d. Reported suicide rates are probably lower than actual rate.

3/23   c
          Mood Disorders
          Page #43

Which statement is most accurate regarding the relationship between sex and suicide?

a. Men and women attempt suicide at about the same rate.
b. Men and women commit suicide at at about the same rate.
c. Men commit suicide more often than women, but women attempt suicide more often than men.
d. Women commit suicide more often than men, but men attempt suicide more often than women.

3/24   d
          Mood Disorders
          Pages #43-44

Which of the following sets of warning signs is the best indicator of suicide risk?

a. fear of dying, shortness of breath, a feeling of unreality, sweating
b. aggressive behavior, acting out, periods of intense anger, agitation
c. loss of ability to think clearly, hallucinations, fear of other people
d. verbal or behavioral clues, dramatic changes in routine, depression

3/25   a
          Anxiety Disorders
          Page #45

Which of the following statements about phobias is most accurate?

a. Phobias are the most common anxiety disorder.
b. A phobia is marked by excessive or unrealistic worry lasting 6 months or longer.
c. The causes of phobias are quite well understood.
d. Most phobias do not respond to treatment.

3/26   c
        Anxiety Disorders
        Page #44

The primary difference between general anxiety and a panic attack is

a. panic attacks cause physiological responses and anxiety doesn't.
b. panic attacks usually occur during the day, general anxiety at night.
c. the intensity and sudden onset of the symptoms.
d. their differing effects on men and women.

3/27   c
        Personality Disorders
        Page #46

Personality disorders include paranoia, obsessive-compulsive personality, and

a. post-traumatic stress disorder
b. schizophrenia
c. narcissism
d. suicide.

3/28   d
        Eating Disorders
        Page #46

The two most prevalent forms of eating disorders are

a. bulimia nervosa and narcissism.
b. bulimarexia and anemia.
c. anorexia nervosa and obesity.
d. anorexia nervosa and bulimia nervosa.

3/29   b
        Personality Disorders
        Page #46

Paranoia is defined as the tendency to

a. to be preoccupied with details and routines.
b. view the actions of others as deliberately threatening or annoying.
c. have false beliefs regarding oneself or the world.
d. be oversensitive to criticisms or suggestions.

3/30   c
        Eating Disorders
        Page #47

Which of the following statements about anorexia nervosa is most accurate?

a. It is primarily an appetite disturbance.
b. It rarely causes death.
c. It is primarily a female disorder.
d. Victims are mostly lower-class women in their mid-thirties.

3/31   a
Eating Disorders
Pages #47-48

Which of the following symptoms is common to both anorexia and bulimia nervosa?

a. overconcern with weight and body image
b. loss of menstrual cycle
c. binge eating
d. "traditional" family background

3/32   d
Schizophrenic Disorders
Page #50

Schizophrenic disorders are characterized by a highly distorted sense of

a. internal reality.
b. moral reality.
c. external reality.
d. external and internal reality.

3/33   c
Schizophrenic Disorders
Page #50

Which of the following statements is not true? Schizophrenic disorders

a. impair thinking and speech.
b. occur everywhere in the world.
c. affects mostly older adults.
d. have mild to severe symptoms.

3/34   b
Schizophrenic Disorders
Page #50

The primary symptoms of schizophrenia include hallucinations, delusions, and

a. flashbacks.
b. thought disorders.
c. violent behavior.
d. split personality.

3/35   a
Finding Help
Page #52

Most people who seek help from mental health professionals have problems that are

a. related to current stresses or rooted in the past.
b. related to a personal weakness or lack of character.
c. shizophrenic in nature.
d. unrelated to the present and caused by childhood trauma.

3/36   d
Therapy
Page #54

Psychoanalysis, a form of psychodynamic therapy pioneered by Freud, emphasizes the importance of

a. psychic experiences.
b. stress and disease.
c. behavior over feelings.
d. early childhood events.

3/37   c
Recovery
Page #57

Mental illness should <u>not</u> be considered

a. normal, like physical illness.
b. to have specific beginning and end-
   ing points.
c. immoral or bizarre.
d. a temporary abnormality.

Matching

3/38   Directions: Match each of the levels of Menninger's continuum on the
left with its correct description on the right. Each set of
descriptors may be used only once.

<u>Level</u>

<u>Descriptors</u>

1. __ Level 1
2. __ Level 2
3. __ Level 3
4. __ Level 4
5. __ Level 5

a. social offenses, open aggression,
   violent acts
b. personality disorders, phobias
c. severe psychological deterioration,
   loss of will to live
d. Hyperreactions, anxiety, nervous-
   ness, minor physical symptoms
e. normal coping devices and ego
   control
f. severe depression, psychotic and
   bizarre behavior

1-d, 2-b, 3-a, 4-f, 5-c
Mental Illness
Page #35

3/39   Directions: Match each of the mental disorders on the left with its
        correct set of symptoms on the right. Each set of symptoms may only
        be used once.

	Disorder	Symptoms
1.	__ Depression	a. perception of sights or sounds not actually present
2.	__ Phobia	b. gross impairment in perception of reality
3.	__ Paranoia	c. a false belief about one's self or the world
4.	__ Anorexia Nervosa	d. an exaggerated and persistent fear
5.	__ Bulimia Nervosa	e. episodic binge eating followed by purge vomiting
6.	__ Delusion	f. unexpected and intense experiences of fear and terror
7.	__ Hallucination	g. refusal to eat, or lack of eating resulting in malnutrition
		h. perceiving other's actions to be threatening or demeaning
		i. feelings of unhappiness and despair

    1-i, 2-d, 3-h, 4-g, 5-e, 6-c, 7-a
    Mental Illness
    Pages #38-50

Completion

3/40   * feeling sad and hopeless   Identify three of the five criteria
        * loss of interest/pleasure   used to diagnose depression.
        * loss of weight/appetite   1. _____
        * sleep disorders, agitation   2. _____
        * fatigue/thoughts of death   3. _____
        * impaired thinking ability
        * feelings of guilt or
          worthlessness

        Mood Disorders
        Page #39

3/41   * Listen sympathetically.   Identify three things you can do to
        * Be honest about your con-   help someone you care about who's de-
          cerns.   pressed.
        * Discuss probable causes.   1. _____
        * Keep your friend active.   2. _____
        * Watch for any hint of   3. _____
          suicidal intention.
        * Don't dismiss their fears.

        Mood Disorders
        Page #42

3/42
* increased moodiness
* depression
* threats of suicide
* isolation
* changes in personal habits
* recent failures or failed relationships
* cheerfulness after a depression
* giving away favorite possessions
* withdrawal

Mood Disorders
Pages #43-44

Identify five warning signals for suicide.
1. _____
2. _____
3. _____
4. _____
5. _____

3/43
* talk it out/listen
* suggest solutions,
* ask directly about intentions of suicide
* take threats seriously
* get help if you get stuck
* stay close until help arrives
* if you must leave your friend alone, get them to promise they won't do anything hurtful/harmful without calling you first

Mood Disorders
Page #44

Identify four strategies you can use with someone you know to prevent suicide.
1. _____
2. _____
3. _____
4. _____

3/44
* sudden or severe change of weight
* solitary dining
* frequent nausea or constipation
* excessive fear of weight gain
* menstrual irregularities
* food hoarding
* meal skipping

Eating Disorders
Pages #47-48

What are three warning signs of eating disorders?
1. _____
2. _____
3. _____

3/45
* prolonged depression
* thoughts of suicide
* problems with sleeping, relationships or sex
* violent or destructive behavior
* a sense that your life is out of control
* impaired thinking ability
* problems with alcohol

Finding Help
Page #51

Identify four signs of trouble that signal a need for help from a mental health professional.
1. _____
2. _____
3. _____
4. _____

3/46
* get information about fees and schedules
* check on credentials
* find out about patients with similar problems
* consider your intuitive reaction to the therapist and the environment
* if you are not satisfied, ask for a referral to another therapist

Finding Help
Page #55

What are five considerations important to the choosing of a therapist?
1. _____
2. _____
3. _____
4. _____
5. _____

3/47
* learn as much as you can about the illness
* seek help if you are unable to cope
* understand and monitor medication
* don't abandon the person

Recovery
Page #59

Identify three things you could do if a loved one developed a mental disorder.
1. _____
2. _____
3. _____

Essay

3/48   Is mental illness culturally defined, or are there standards for mental health that apply in widely divergent cultures? What information do you have to support your point of view?

3/49   If you were suffering from a mental disorder, where would you go for treatment? Discuss the advantages and disadvantages of the various facilities and personnel who treat the mentally ill. Based on the quality of care available, do you think our society has overcome its bias against mental illness? Why, or why not?

3/50   Exercise and physical activity is now being recognized as helpful in the treatment of certain types of mental disorders. What does physical fitness have to do with mental health? Do you think diet might have a similar role? Why, or why not?

Section I - Your Mind: The Quest for Understanding

Chapter 4: Stress

In this chapter -

* Stress
* Stressors
* Effects of Stress
* Prevention
* Stress Management

Section I - Your Mind: The Quest for Understanding
Chapter 4: Stress

True-False

4/1   True
       Stress
       Page #61

An individual's response to a stressful situation is what determines its
physical and psychological impact.

4/2   False
       Stress
       Page #61

Stress is avoidable.

4/3   True
       Stress
       Page #61

According to Dr. Hans Selye, stress is
defined as the response of the body to
any demand made upon it.

4/4   True
       Stress
       Page #61

Stress is essential to survival.

4/5   False
       Stressors
       Page #64

Life changes are rarely associated with
stress.

4/6   True
       Stressors
       Page # 69

Burn-out refers to a state of physical,
mental, and emotional exhaustion
brought about by emotional pressure.

4/7   False
       Effects of Stress
       Page #69

There is very little, if any, evidence
to indicate that stress is related to
physical disease.

4/8   False
       Effects of Stress
       Page #70

The Type-B behavior pattern is characterized by an aggressive approach to
work and success.

4/9   True
       Effects of Stress
       Page #70

In one research study, the Type-A
behavior pattern was the major
contributing factor to the early development of coronary artery disease.

4/10   False
       Effects of Stress
       Page #71

Migraine headaches are caused by the
involuntary contraction of the scalp,
neck, and head muscles.

4/11   True
       Prevention
       Page #74

Adaptation, a change in structure,
form, or behavior to suit a new situation, is a positive response to stress.

Chapter 4: Stress

4/12   True
        Stress Management
        Page #76

Research indicates that biofeedback, hypnosis, and meditation are all effective in reducing high blood pressure.

Mulitple Choice

4/13   a
        Stress
        Page # 61

Eustress is

a. positive stress that stimulates healthy functioning.
b. negative stress that may cause illness.
c. the first stage of the General Adaptation Syndrome.
d. a non-specific response of the body to demands placed upon it.

4/14   c
        Stress
        Pages #61-63

The General Adaptation Syndrome, or G.A.S., consists of three stages. What are they?

a. distress, adaptation, and homeostasis
b. stress, alarm, and resistance
c. alarm, resistance, and exhaustion
d. eustress, distress, and homeostasis

4/15   d
        Stress
        Page #63

Which of the following is not a signal of stress overload?

a. physical symptoms like fatigue, headaches, or diarrhea
b. problems with concentration
c. overuse of non-prescription drugs
d. aggressive or competitive behavior

4/16   b
        Effects of Stress
        Pages #69-72

Which of the following statements about the effect of stress is most accurate?

a. Blood pressure changes and stress response are unrelated.
b. Chemicals triggered by the stress response suppress the immune system.
c. Stress causes ulcers.
d. The role of stress in personal health is minor.

4/17   b
        Prevention
        Pages #72-75

Which of the following is most effective in preventing stress?

a. eliminating stressors from your life
b. adopting a flexible and positive attitude toward unplanned changes
c. working alone to take care of yourself.
d. waiting until the situation changes

4/18   a
        Stress Management
        Pages #76-80

Effective techniques for managing stress include relaxation, meditation, biofeedback, and

a. exercise.
b. Type-A behavior.
c. avoiding strong feelings.
d. aspirin.

4/19   c
        Stress
        Page #62

Which of the following statements about the General Adaptation Syndrome is most accurate?

a. The stages of the G.A.S. occur in different order depending on the stressor involved.
b. The most pronounced physical changes occur during the resistance stage.
c. During the exhaustion stage, the physical signs of the first stage (alarm) reappear.
d. The "fight or flight" mechanism is activated during the resistance stage.

4/20   a
        Stress
        Page #61

Which of the following statements about stress is most accurate?

a. Stress is essential to survival.
b. Stress is really nervous tension.
c. Stress is harmful to the body.
d. Stress should be totally avoided.

4/21   c
        Stressors
        Pages #65-66

Which of the following strategies is most effective for coping with change?

a. Focus on your own problems.
b. Don't confuse physical complaints with the stress of change.
c. Set a balanced routine of work and recreation.
d. Regard your problems seriously, don't laugh at them.

4/22   d
        Stressors
        Page #67

Daily hassles identified as most
disturbing include losing things,
trying to look better physically, and

a. being bored.
b. not having enough money.
c. violent confrontations.
d. having too much to do.

4/23   a
        Stressors
        Page #68

Which of the following statements about
work and stress is most accurate?

a. Rises in the rate of unemployment
   are correlated with rises in suicide
   rates.
b. Workaholics are characterized by the
   inefficient use of time.
c. One sign of burn-out is increased
   interest in sex.
d. Mixing your personal and work life
   can prevent burn-out.

4/24   c
        Effects of Stress
        Page #70

Research on stress and sudden death
indicates that

a. stress causes sudden death.
b. bad news triggers sudden death, but
   good news does not.
c. sudden death is often preceeded by
   a series of life changes.
d. the "fight or flight" response is
   responsible for sudden death.

4/25   b
        Effects of Stress
        Page #71

Under which of the following conditions
does immune suppression occur?

a. during meditation
b. following traumatic stress
c. during migraine headaches
d. just prior to coronary artery
   disease

4/26   d
        Effects of Stress
        Page #69

Which statement most accurately states
the relationship between stress and
the body.

a. Of all the complications associated
   with stress, sudden death is the
   most serious.
b. Counseling is ineffective in changing Type-A behavior patterns.
c. Stress affects only certain organ
   systems in the body.
d. Stress is considered by many to be
   our number one health enemy.

4/27   c
        Prevention
        Page #73

Characteristics of stress-resistant
personalities include a commitment to
self, work, and family; a sense of
control over one's life; and

a. a belief in psychosomatic illness.
b an understanding of the difference
   between eustress and distress.
c. the ability to see change as a
   challenge.
d. the desire to avoid stress.

4/28   a
        Prevention
        Page #73

Which of the following is not one of
the three types of daily stress
situations described by David Elkind?

a. not forseeable, but avoidable
b. forseeable and avoidable
c. neither forseeable nor avoidable
d. forseeable but not avoidable

4/29   b
        Prevention
        Pages #76-77

Some of the benefits of stress
prevention strategies include improved
immune responses, sense of self-worth,
and

a. reduced adaptation.
b. increased altruistic egotism.
c. decreased altruistic egotism.
d. increased general adaptation
   syndrome.

4/30   c
        Prevention
        Pages #74-75

Which of the following is not an
effective strategy for preventing
stress?

a. keeping a stress diary
b. developing positive feelings
c. using non-prescription medicine
d. coming to terms with your life

4/31   d
        Prevention
        Page #76

The best personal strategy for
handling stress is to

a. avoid hassles by avoiding other
   people.
b. focus on a project or work when
   you get tired of dealing with a
   problem.
c. identify people who are causing you
   stress.
d. develop adaptative responses to
   stressors.

4/32   b
        Stress Management
        Pages #76-80

Most approaches to stress management
focus on

a. proper balance of medication.
b. your ability to control your own
   response to stress.
c. "new age" techniques with little or
   or no proven effectiveness.
d. visualization as the single best
   technique.

4/33   c
        Stress Management
        Page #77

Which of the following statements about
relaxation is most accurate?

a. It is most effective immediately
   following a meal.
b. It produces a state of eustress.
c. It enhances immune functioning.
d. It does not affect mental activity.

4/34   d
        Stress Managemente
        Pages #79-80

Effective techniques for stress
management include meditation, biofeedback, relaxation, and

a. Type-A behavior.
b. Type-B behavior.
c. anaerobic exercise.
d. aerobic exercise.

4/35   b
        Stress Management
        Page #79

Biofeedback is a learning process used
to manage stress that includes developing increased awareness of the body,
gaining control over it, and

a. learning to use an electronic feedback device in everyday living.
b. transferring control to everyday
   living.
c. permanently changing blood pressure
   heart rate levels.
d. reducing the brain's alpha wave
   output.

Matching

4/36   Directions: Match each step of Herbert Benson's Relaxation Response technique on the left with its correct corresponding activity on the right. Each activity description may be used only once, **and all activities must be listed in their proper sequence (eg, step #1 first, step #2 second, and so on).**

	Steps (in sequence)
1.	__ First Step
2.	__ Second Step
3.	__ Third Step
4.	__ Fourth Step
5.	__ Fifth Step
6.	__ Sixth Step

Activity

a. Deeply relax all your muscles, beginning at your feet and progressing to your face.
b. Continue the breathing pattern for 10 to 20 minutes.
c. Close your eyes.
d. Imagine something that worries or scares you.
e. Sit quietly in a comfortable position.
f. Breathe through your nose; say "one" silently at the end of each exhale.
g. Visualize yourself exhaling tension and stress during each exhale.
h. Allow distracting thoughts to disappear on their own, and return to your breathing.

1-e, 2-c, 3-a,
4-f, 5-b, 6-h
Prevention
Page #77

4/37   Directions: Match each stress-related concept on the left with
        correct definition on the right. Each definition may be used only
        once.

            Concept   Definition

1. __ homeostasis   a. the first stage of the General
2. __ distress   Adaptation Response
3. __ stressor   b. agents or situations that trigger
4. __ eustress   the body's stress response
5. __ stress   c. the body's natural state of
6. __ psychosomatic   balance or stability
                              d. physical illness caused by psycho-
                                 logical factors
                              e. the response of the body to demands
                                 placed upon it
                              f. positive stress
                              g. negative stress
                              h. neutral stress

        1-c, 2-g, 3-b,
        4-f, 5-e, 6-d
        Stress
        Pages #61-70

Completion

4/38   * alarm   Which two stages of the General
        * exhaustion   Adaptation Syndrome are marked by
        Stress   abnormal physical symptoms.
        Page #61   1. _____
                                 2. _____

4/39   * Seek accurate data about   Identify three things you can do to
          what's happening in your   cope with change in your life.
          life.   1. _____
        * Tune in to your body.   2. _____
        * Balance work and recrea-   3. _____
          tion.
        * Share your worries.
        Stressors
        Page #65

4/40   time management   Alf keeps a daily "to-do list, has
        Stressors   learned to say "no", divides large
        Page #67   tasks into smaller ones, and rewards
                                 himself when he completes a part.
                                 What strategy is Alf using to control
                                 stress?

                                 _____

4/41 * describing stressful situations and your reactions to them
      * identifying ways of preventing stressful reactions
      * analyzing your relationships with people who trigger your stress reactions.
      * eliminating unimportant commitments
      Prevention
      Page #74

Name three activities associated with keeping a stress diary.
1. _____
2. _____
3. _____

4/42 laughter/humor
      Prevention
      Page #75

In his book, <u>Anatomy of an Illness as Perceived by the Patient</u>, author Norman Cousins describes an uncommon approach to healing and recovery. What is it?

_____

4/43 * breathing
      * visualization/imagery
      * relaxation
      Stress Management
      Pages #76-80

What are the three basic components of most approaches to stress management?
1. _____
2. _____
3. _____

4/44 Biofeedback
      Stress Management
      Page #79

Martha is learning to stimulate her brain's production of alpha waves. Which method of stress management is she using?

_____

4/45
      * physical symtoms
      * frequent illness
      * problems with studies or work
      * extreme behavior
      * bizarre behavior
      * becoming accident-prone.
      * overuse of self medications
      * overwork
      * denial
      * isolation
      Stress
      Page #63

Identify five warning signals of stress overload.
1. _____
2. _____
3. _____
4. _____
5. _____

Essay

4/46   "Belief in your ability to control your response to stress is the single most powerful tool you have in defending yourself against the negative impact of stress." Do you agree with this statement? If so, why? If not, why not? Use examples to support your point of view.

4/47   Briefly describe a recent stressful experience in your life using the framework of the General Adaptation Syndrome (eg, the stages of alarm, resistance, and exhaustion). Incorporate the following terms into your description:

   stressor(s)
   eustress/distress
   homeostasis
   adaptive response

4/48   Describe the role that early childhood experiences and attitudes play in the development of our response to stress.

4/49   If you were in a position to legislate reforms that would reduce the level of stress in our society, what changes would you mandate? Defend your decisions using the following criteria:

   - the proposed changes don't benefit one group at the expense of another
   - the long-term impact of the changes does not result in increased levels of stress for major population groups
   - the proposed changes don't adversely affect the economy

4/50   Develop a stress-prevention/stress-management program for yourself. Describe the components of the program, what you hope to achieve, and a schedule for implementation.

<u>AN INVITATION TO HEALTH</u>
TEST BANK

Section II - Your Body: A Lifetime of Wellness

<u>Chapter 5: Nutrition</u>

In this chapter -

* Nutrients
* Four Food Groups
* Prevention
* Myths and Controversies

Section II - Your Body: A Lifetime of Wellness
Chapter 5: Nutrition

True-False

5/1	True Nutrients Page #87	The interaction between a living organism and its food is the focus of nutrition.
5/2	False Nutrients Page #87	The first step in the digestive process is primarily chemical in nature.
5/3	False Nutrients Page #87	Not everyone needs the same basic nutrients.
5/4	True Nutrients Page #87	The basic components of proteins are amino acids.
5/5	False Nutrients Page #89	Ideally, complex carbohydrates, or starches, should comprise about 25% of the daily calories in our diet.
5/6	True Nutrients Page #92	Water-soluble vitamins must be replaced daily.
5/7	True Four Food Groups Page #94	No single food provides all the nutrients, vitamins, and protein your body needs.
5/8	False Prevention Page #99	Recent research has shown that our diet does not affect the risk of contracting cancer and heart disease.
5/9	True Prevention Page #100	For adults over 20, it is recommended that total cholesterol be below 200 mg per deciliter of blood (200 mg/dl).
5/10	True Prevention Page #103	No single food has been found to be effective in preventing cancer.
5/11	False Myths and Controversies Page #107	Nutritional controversies are most effectively resolved using a single research approach called epidemiology.

5/12   False
            Myths and Controversies
            Page #110

Vitamin C has been proven effective in preventing the common cold.

Multiple Choice

5/13   c
            Nutrients
            Page #87

Essential nutrients include proteins, fats, vitamins, minerals, and

a. fiber.
b. cholesterol.
c. carbohydrates.
d. amino acids.

5/14   a
            Nutrients
            Page #88

Which of the following statements about protein is most accurate?

a. Most Americans consume about twice as much protein as they need.
b. An essential amino acid is one which the human body can produce itself.
c. Incomplete proteins are missing some essential saturated fats.
d. 25% of your daily calories should come from protein.

5/15   d
            Page #90

Functions of fat include storing vita- from shock or extreme temperatures, and

a. maintaining eyesight.
b. cleaning the blood.
c. stimulating the heart.
d. keeping our skin healthy.

5/16   d
            Nutrients
            Page #94

The two important minerals that most people do not get enough of are

a. gold and lead.
b. zinc and cobalt.
c. chlorine and iodine.
d. iron and calcium.

5/17   a
            Four Food Groups
            Pages #97-99

The Basic Four Food Groups are fruit and vegetables, bread and cereals, milk and cheese, and

a. meat, poultry, and fish.
b. fast foods.
c. alcohol, snacks, and desserts.
d. fiber and organic foods.

5/18   d
        Prevention
        Page #100

According to the National Heart, Lung, and Blood Institute, a 1 percent drop in blood cholesterol level causes the risk of heart attack to

a. increase by 2 percent.
b. increase by 5 percent.
c. decrease by 5 percent.
d. decrease by 2 percent.

5/19   d
        Prevention
        Page #100

The blood cholesterol level at which the risk of heart disease is dangerously high and strict dietary changes are recommended is

a. 200 mg/dl.
b. 220 mg/dl.
c. 230 mg/dl.
d. 240 mg/dl.

5/20   b
        Prevention
        Page #102

Which of the following statements about fish is <u>least</u> accurate?

a. Americans eat, on the average, about 13 pounds of fish per year.
b. Omega-3 fatty acids, found in fish oils, are saturated fats.
c. Recent research shows that two fish meals per week can reduce the risk of heart attack by 50 percent.
d. Omega-3 fatty acids change the chemistry of the blood.

5/21   c
        Prevention
        Page #104

The impact of diet on cancer rates has focused primarily on the intake of

a. meat and alcohol.
b. vitamins and minerals.
c. fat and fiber.
d. free radicals.

5/22   c
        Myths and Controversies
        Page #107

Which of the following statements most accurately reflects current research on sugar?

a. There is a positive correlation between sugar intake and heart disease.
b. Sugar intake contributes to behavior disorders.
c. <u>How</u> you eat sugar impacts your dental health more than how <u>much</u> sugar you eat.
d. Insulin is produced by the pancreas when blood sugar levels are low.

5/23   d
Myths and Controversies
Page #108

Fiber is

a. high in calories.
b. found primarily in animal products.
c. nutritious.
d. effective in preventing inflammation of the bowel.

5/24   a.
Myths and Controversies
Page #108

Which of the following statements about caffeine is most accurate?

a. Caffeine is the world's most used drug.
b. Excessive caffeine consumption has been shown to cause cancer.
c. The average American drinks 82 gallons of coffee per year.
d. Caffeine does not cross the placenta into the tissues of a fetus.

5/25   c.
Myths and Controversies
Page #110

Research now shows that moderate doses of Vitamin C can

a. prevent the common cold.
b. cure asthma.
c. help prevent iron deficiency anemia.
d. reverse atherosclerosis (narrowing of the arteries).

5/26   b
Myths and Controversies
Page #113

Which of the following is not an artificial sweetener?

a. aspartame
b. phenylketonuria
c. saccharin
d. NutraSweet

5/27   c
Nutrients
Page #87

Most digestion and absorption take place in the

a. large intestine.
b. stomach.
c. small intestine.
d. mouth during chewing.

5/28   a
Nutrients
Page #87

The amount of basic nutrients required by an individual depends on his/her sex, size, health,

a. age, and level of activity.
b. race, and amount of vitamin supplements taken.
c. blood type, and weight.
d. attitude, and level of fitness.

5/29   b
Nutrients
Page #89

Which of the following combinations of
foods does not provide complete protein?

a. soy and rice
b. tortillas and rice
c. beans and rice
d. sesame and chick-peas

5/30   d
Nutrients
Page #89

The advantage of complex carbohydrates
(starches) over simple carbohydrates
(sugars) is that starches

a. have more fiber.
b. have more protein.
c. have fewer calories per gram.
d. have more nutrients.

5/31   c
Nutrients
Page #91

Which of the following statements about
cholesterol is most accurate?

a. Cholesterol levels in the blood are
   related to the consumption of un-
   saturated fats.
b. Cholesterol cannot be produced by
   the body.
c. Cholesterol is necessary for liver
   functioning.
d. Elevated cholesterol levels in the
   blood cause obesity.

5/32   d
Nutrients
Page #96

Which of the following strategies is
least effective in increasing the
amount of iron in your diet?

a. Eat more legumes, fresh fruits,
   whole grain cereals and broccoli.
b. Eat more lean, red meat.
c. Combine foods high in iron with
   those high in Vitamin C to increase
   absorption.
d. Combine foods high in iron with tea
   to increase absorption.

5/33   b
Prevention
Page #102

Which of the following uses of red
meat is most effective in reducing
the risk of heart disease?

a. Fry red meat whenever possible.
b. Limit red meat servings to two
   or three per week, with servings
   between 2 and 3 ounces.
c. Use salt to tenderize red meat.
d. Baste red meat with its own
   drippings.

5/34   b
       Prevention
       Page #103

In order to safely increase your consumption of Omega-3 fatty acids, you
should

a. take fish oil supplements.
b. substitute cold water ocean fish
   for meat.
c. fry the fish you eat.
d. increase your consumption of processed fish.

5/35   a
       Prevention
       Page #103

Harold is interested in reducing his
intake of salt. For best results, he
should

a. choose processed foods that are
   low in sodium.
b. top using salt altogether - go
   "cold turkey."
c. wait until his blood pressure begins
   to rise, and then cut back.
d. use no salt during cooking, and
   limit himself to salt at the table.

5/36   c
       Prevention
       Page #106

Which statement best describes the
relationship between diet and cancer.

a. Excess dietary fat causes cancer.
b. Insufficient dietary fiber causes
   cancer.
c. Cruciferous vegetables (such as
   broccoli) are effective against
   certain kinds of pre-cancerous
   molecules called free radicals.
d. Eating foods high in vitamins C
   and E promotes free radicals in
   the body.

5/37   a
       Myths and Controversies
       Page #107

Sean wants to cut down on his sugar
intake. He should

a. choose fruit instead of candy.
b. change from white sugar to brown
   sugar.
c. limit sweets to between-meal
   snacks.
d. keep only the amount of dessert
   on-hand that he will need for
   entertaining.

5/38   c
Myths and Controversies
Page #110

Which of the following statements about fast food is most accurate?

a. Pizza is low in essential nutrients.
b. Most fast food "shakes" are made with milk.
c. Fast foods tend to be high in fat and sodium.
d. Fast foods tend to be high in fiber.

5/39   b
Myths and Controversies
Pages #111-112

Celeste is thinking about eating more organic food. Before switching, she should realize that

a. organic food is generally cheaper than non-organic food.
b. there is no basis for claiming that organic food has more food value.
c. the terms "natural" and "health" have been given very specific meanings by the Food and Drug Administration.
d. granola is low in fat and calories.

5/40   d
Myths and Controversies
Page #113

You're shopping for a nutritious brand of crackers, and begin to read the food label of a box you've selected. It says: "Measurable amounts of important nutrients." What this means is

a. recommended daily requirements of essential vitamins and minerals.
b. recommended daily requirements of protein and carbohydrates.
c. at least 10 percent of the recommended daily requirement of some nutrients.
d. at least 2 percent of the recommended daily requirement of some nutrients.

Matching

5/41   Directions: Match each of the food groups on the left with the
        correct set of nutritional benefits on the right. Each set of
        benefits may only be used once.

	Food Group	Benefits
1.	__ Vegetables and Fruit	a. high in calcium, riboflavin, protein, and vitamins A and B
2.	__ Bread and Cereal	b. low in fat, high in fiber, and contribute vitamins A and C
3.	__ Milk and Cheese	c. high in calories, low in fiber, some minerals
4.	__ Meat/Fish/Poultry/Beans	d. high in protein, phosphorous, iron, zinc, and vitamin B
		e. important source of B vitamins, iron, protein, and fiber

1-b, 2-e, 3-a, 4-d
Four Food Groups
Pages #97-99

5/42   Directions: Match each of the basic nutrients on the left with its
        correct physiological function on the right. Each function may be
        used only once.

	Nutrient	Function(s)
1.	__ Protein	a. provides body and brain with glucose (sugar), vitamins and minerals
2.	__ Fats	b. store vitamins, maintain skin, provide stamina, protect against shock
3.	__ Carbohydrates	c. essential for utilizing protein, fats, and carbohydrates; make blood cells and hormones
4.	__ Vitamins	d. framework for muscle, bones, hair, blood, and tissue repair
5.	__ Minerals	e. used to assist digestion and transportation of nutrients
		f. used for building bones and teeth, aid in muscle and nervous system operation

1-d, 2-b, 3-a, 4-c, 5-f
Nutrients
Pages #87-90

Completion

5/43   * protein
        * carbohydrates
        * fats
        * vitamins
        * minerals

        Nutrients
        Page #87

Identify the five categories of basic nutrients.
1. _____
2. _____
3. _____
4. _____
5. _____

5/44   * cholesterol
        Nutrients
        Page #100

Health risks associated with the increased intake of saturated fats are due to increases in the blood level of

_____.

5/45   * two
        Nutrients
        Page #91

How many cups of water should you drink for every pound of weight loss due to hard work, play, or exercise?

_____

5/46   * increase consumption of
          dairy products
        * increase consumption of
          other calcium-rich foods
          like sardines or tofu
        * eat foods rich in vitamin
          C at the same time
        * use acidic dressing to
          increase calcium absorp-
          tion from salad greens
        * use supplements, but not
          those made from dolomite
          or bone meal
        Nutrients
        Page #97

Identify three things you can do to increase the amount of calcium in your diet.
1. _____
2. _____
3. _____

5/47   * cut total fat to 30 per-
          cent of daily calories
        * keep saturated fat below
          10 percent if possible.
        * keep polyunsaturated fats
          below 10 percent of daily
          diet
        * keep daily cholesterol
          intake to less than 100
          mg per 1,000 calories
        * no more than two alcoholic
          drinks per day
        * limit sodium to no more
          than 1,000 mg per 1,000
          calories, or 3,000 mg
          per day
        Prevention
        Page #99

Identify four recommendations of the American Heart Association for reducing the risk of heart disease.
1. _____
2. _____
3. _____
4. _____

5/48

* cut fat to 30 percent
  of daily calories
* increase fiber intake
* drink 2-4 glasses of milk
  per day or take calcium
  supplements
* eat fish twice a week
* eat vegetables two or
  three times per day
* make sure you're eating
  foods that supply enough
  vitamin A and C
* increase amount of vitamin
  E in your daily diet
* increase amount of selenium
  in your diet
* get enough folic acid
* eat hamburger rare or
  medium; don't fry, barbeque
  or grill hamburger
* limit smoked or processed
  foods
* no more than two alcoholic
  drinks per day

Prevention
Pages #105-107

Identify five recommendations for an anti-cancer diet.

1. _____
2. _____
3. _____
4. _____
5. _____

5/49

* lower incidence of colon
  and breast cancer
* lower incidence of heart
  disease
* lower incidence of osteoporosis

Myths and Controversies
Page #112

Identify two advantages of a vegetarian diet.

1. _____
2. _____

5/50

* eat a variety of foods
* maintain desirable weight
* avoid too much fat
* get enough starch and
  fiber
* avoid too much sugar
* avoid too much sodium
* drink alcohol only in
  moderation

Prevention
Page #116

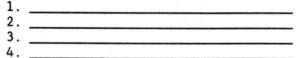

Identify four of the dietary guidelines for Americans developed by the US Department of Agriculture and Department of Health and Human Services.

1. _____
2. _____
3. _____
4. _____

Essay

5/51   Think about the last food item you ate (eg, such as a sandwich, bowl of cereal, salad, or candy bar). Describe what happened to that food item from the time it entered your mouth until it was metabolized by your body. Be sure to include the following in your dicussion:

- elements of the digestive process
- nutritional components and functions of the food you ate
- the benefits and risks (if any) of what you ate
- the probable long-term effect on your body of the food you ate

5/52   Defend or attack the following statement:

"The price of food should be determined by its nutritional value; unprocessed foods high in nutrients and low in fats or other additives should be cheapest, and processed or fast/junk foods should be the most expensive."

What would happen to our eating habits if this were true? What would happen to the food industry in this country?

5/53   Take a look at your own diet, and prescribe at least five changes that would have a beneficial effect on your health. For each change you propose, describe briefly how you might actually implement the improvement. Make a copy of your answer to this question, and give it to a friend. Ask them to help you make the changes.

5/54   What changes have you seen or heard about in the fast food industry that occurred as a response to increasing consumer interest in health? Why doesn't the fast food industry take the initiative in promoting good diet and nutrition?

5/55   Identify some of the resources in your community that can provide additional information about diet and nutrition.

Section II - Your Body: A Lifetime of Wellness

<u>Chapter 6: Weight Control</u>

In this chapter -

* Personal Weight
* Calories
* Hunger and Appetite
* Obesity
* Dieting
* Weight Management

Section II - Your Body: A Lifetime of Wellness
Chapter 6: Weight Control

True-False

6/1   True
Personal Weight
Page #120

Most Americans are fat because they eat too much and exercise too little.

6/2   False
Personal Weight
Page #122

Low-carbohydrate dieting is an effective method for achieving sustained weight loss.

6/3   False
Calories
Page #124

Consuming excess calories in the form of fatty foods results in more body fat than consuming the same number of excess calories as protein or carbohydrates.

6/4   True
Hunger and Appetite
Page #130

Satiety is the feeling of fullness and relief from hunger.

6/5   False
Hunger and Appetite
Page #127

Your blood sugar level is the main determinant of your appetite level.

6/6   True
Obesity
Page #131

According to the text's definition of obesity, it is possible to be overweight without being obese.

6/7   True
Obesity
Page #131

Obesity is strongly correlated with the weights of a person's biological parents.

6/8   False
Dieting
Page #132

Most diets fail because the people who try them aren't really motivated to lose weight.

6/9   False
Dieting
Pages #134-135

Fasting is an effective method for losing weight.

6/10   True
Weight Management
Page #138

The secret of permanent weight control is adhering to a lifelong program of sensible eating and exercise.

Chapter 6: Weight Control

<u>Multiple Choice</u>

6/11   c
Personal Weight
Page #120

The percentage of adult Americans be-tween the ages of 25 and 74 who are overweight is approximately

a. 8 percent.
b. 18 percent.
c. 28 percent.
d. 38 percent.

6/12   a
Personal Weight
Page #120

Which of the following statements about personal weight in America is most accurate?

a. Slimness is often associated with glamour, success, and happiness.
b. Overweight people lack willpower.
c. Chronic dieting is quite rare.
d. Social pressure does not play a significant role in determining our attitudes toward personal weight.

6/13   d
Personal Weight
Page #122

Your personal weight is determined by your eating behavior, food selection, amount of daily exercise, and your

a. age.
b. self concept.
c. income level.
d. genetic makeup.

6/14   c
Calories
Page #124

On the average, Americans consume 3,300 calories per day - enough to support an active person who weighs at least

a. 150 pounds.
b. 170 pounds.
c. 190 pounds.
d. 210 pounds.

6/15   b
Hunger and Appetite
Page #127

Hunger is

a. the fear of not having food.
b. the physiological drive to consume food.
c. determined by stomach contractions.
d. unrelated to chemical activity in the brain.

6/16

b
Hunger and Appetite
Pages #128-129

Your appetite is sensitive to the type
of food available, sensual pleasure of
eating, childhood learning, and your

a. height.
b. level of stress.
c. ideal weight range.
d. age.

6/17   a
Hunger and Appetite
Page #131

Set-point theory holds that our bodies
regulate our appetite in order to
insure a relatively constant level of

a. body fat.
b. muscle mass.
c. vitamins and minerals.
d. blood sugar.

6/18   c
Obesity
Page #131

Which of the following statements about
obesity in the American population is
most accurate?

a. Obesity decreases with age.
b. There are more obese men than women.
c. There are 11 million moderately
   obese Americans.
d. Obesity is inherited.

6/19   d
Obesity
Page #132

The dangers of obesity are

a. limited to the severely obese.
b. strictly physical.
c. not sufficient to influence life
   expectancy.
d. pervasive in many systems of the
   body.

6/20   c
Dieting
Page #136

The risks of fad diets include

a. water retention.
b. increased metabolic rate.
c. heart failure.
d. vitamin and mineral overdose.

6/21

a
Dieting
Page #141

The type of diet most effective in
sustaining weight loss is one which

a. has a weight loss goal of one to
   two pounds per week.
b. provides low levels of calories
   and high amounts of protein.
c. includes high levels of vitamin
   and mineral supplements.
d. guarantees to reduce your weight
   to the normal range.

61

6/22   b
        Weight Management
        Page #141

If changing the way you eat is the first step to becoming slimmer, then the second step is

a. joining Weight Watchers.
b. maintaining an appropriate exercise program.
c. reducing your intake of liquids.
d. fasting regularly.

6/23   c
        Personal Weight
        Page #141

In deciding how much you want to weigh, it is important to remember that

a. for every height, there is an ideal weight.
b. you can't be too thin.
c. you must set realistic goals and expectations.
d. your optimal weight range will fall as you get older.

6/24   c
        Personal Weight
        Page #122

The acceptable range of body fat percentage for women is

a. lower than the acceptable range for men.
b. the same as the acceptable range for men.
c. higher than the acceptable range for men.
d. determined by age and height.

6/25   a
        Personal Weight
        Page #121

George is five feet, ten inches tall, and has a medium frame. His ideal weight is about

a. 152-166 pounds.
b. 145-152 pounds.
c. 140-145 pounds.
d. 166-172 pounds.

6/26   b
        Personal Weight
        Page #122

Skin calipers are used to measure

a. muscle tone.
b. body fat.
c. body frame size.
d. water retention.

6/27   d
        Calories
        Page #124

Your basal metabolic rate is the number of calories needed to

a. maintain ideal body weight.
b. sustain your body for one day.
c. raise the temperature of 1 gram of water by 1 degree Celsius.
d. sustain your body at rest.

6/28   **a**
Hunger and Appetite
Page #127

Which of the following statements about hunger/appetite is most accurate?

a. External food cues can trigger chemical changes in the brain.
b. Hunger is determined by one specific signal from the brain.
c. Endorphins alone determine our response to hunger.
d. Satiety is not induced chemically.

6/29   **c**
Hunger and Appetite
Page #127

Appetite usually begins with

a. stomach contractions.
b. elevated blood sugar levels.
c. the expectation that pain (hunger) is on the way.
d. the smell of food.

6/30   **b**
Hunger and Appetite
Page #131

The best method for changing our body's set-point is to

a. eat fewer fatty foods.
b. increase our level of physical activity.
c. participate in hydrostatic immersion.
d. count calories.

6/31   **a**
Obesity
Page #132

Fat cells can

a. increase in size, but not number.
b. increase in number, but not size.
c. increase in both size and number.
d. decrease in number as a result of dieting.

6/32   **d**
Obesity
Page #132

In addition to hereditary influences, obesity can be caused by developmental factors, physical activity, emotional influences, and

a. water retention.
b. heart disease.
c. a preference for high-fat foods.
d. social determinants such as income level or education.

6/33   **c**
Obesity
Page #132

Psychological problems such as irritability, depression, anxiety, and hostility are

a. not associated with obesity.
b. regarded as the cause of obesity.
c. considered consequences of obesity.
d. the result of lack of willpower.

6/34   b
Obesity
Page #133

The best approach to treating obesity is determined by

a. the individual's metabolic rate.
b. the severity of the obesity.
c. the person's ideal weight range.
d. the ratio of body fat to lean muscle mass.

6/35

a
Dieting
Page #134

The Air Force Diet, Dr. Atkin's Diet, and the fructose diet are examples of

a. low-carbohydrate diets.
b. low-protein diets.
c. high-protein diets.
d. diets that prevent ketosis.

6/36   d
Dieting
Page #134

High-carbohydrate, low-protein diets force your

a. body to manufacture protein.
b. kidneys and liver to work harder.
c. body to raise its basal metabolism rate.
d. body to break down muscle tissue.

6/37   c
Dieting
Page #135

Diet aids such as laxatives and diuretics

a. work best when taken over a long period of time.
b. rarely cause health problems.
c. may cause mineral loss and dehydration.
d. reduce the number of fat cells.

6/38   b
Dieting
Page #136

Fad diets are

a. based primarily on medical research.
b. potentially life threatening.
c. not associated with heart failure.
d. equally popular with men and women.

6/39   d
Weight Management
Page #141

In conjunction with a diet, exercise

a. will increase appetite.
b. increases the rate of weight loss.
c. helps to maintain fat stores.
d. helps to maintain weight loss.

6/40   c
Weight Management
Page #138

Ideally, the amount of calories that should come from complex carbohydrates in a weight-reduction eating plan is

a. 30 percent.
b. 40 percent.
c. 50 percent.
d. 60 percent.

Completion

6/41   * hydrostatic immersion
       testing
      Hunger and Appetite
      Page #122

Weighing a person in water to determine their amount of buoyant fat is called
_____.

6/42   * "pre-load" your stomach
       before eating
      * avoid fatty foods
      * save sweets for dessert
      * don't gorge on rich-
       tasting, low-calorie foods
      * hide tempting foods
      * don't skip meals
      * eat at a moderate pace
      Hunger and Appetite
      Page #130

Identify four techniques for lowering your appetite level.
1. _____
2. _____
3. _____
4. _____

6/43   * appetite
      Hunger and Appetite
      Page #131

The body's predetermined level of body fat is enforced by the _____.

6/44   * act as if you're already
       slim
      * focus on the parts of your
       body you like
      * don't put yourself down
      * visualize yourself as slim
      * accept compliments
      * try new activities
      Obesity
      Page #133

Identify three techniques for developing a better body image in preparation for losing weight.
1. _____
2. _____
3. _____

6/45

* request baked or broiled entrees
* request low-calorie salad dressing, or dressing on the side
* request fresh, steamed vegetables without salt or butter
* order an appetizer instead of an entree
* ask for luncheon-sized portions
* split your meal with a friend
* take part of your meal home in a bag

Obesity
Page #134

Identify four strategies to keep down calories when eating out.
1. _____
2. _____
3. _____
4. _____

6/46

* dehydration
* nausea
* vomiting
* dizziness
* fatigue

Dieting
Page #134

Identify three health hazards of ketosis (buildup of fat byproducts in the body) associated with low-carbohydrate diets.
1. _____
2. _____
3. _____

6/47

* surgery to reduce stomach volume
* the "gastric bubble"

Obesity
Page #133

Phil weighs 287 pounds, more than twice his desirable weight. What are the two most common forms of treatment for Phil's life threatening severe obesity?
1. _____
2. _____

6/48

* quick weight loss, mostly water
* lowered basal metabolism
* lowered activity level

* food craving
* mood slump (in the dumps)
* irritability
* feelings of stress

Dieting
Page #136

Identify two physical and two psychological signs of the Yo-Yo Syndrome.
1. _____
2. _____

1. _____
2. _____

6/49 Does it:
* include a selection of nutritious foods?
* emphasize moderate portions?
* use foods easy to find and prepare?
* give enough variety?
* work at home, at work, or during leisure time?
* cost too much?

Dieting
Page #138

Name three things you should know about a weight-reduction plan before starting out.
1. _____
2. _____
3. _____

6/50 keep a food diary
* measure exactly what you eat for a few days
* eat less of your usual foods - eat normal portions only
* only make changes in your habits that you can maintain forever.

Weight Management
Page #138

Identify three things you can do to analyze/improve your eating patterns.
1. _____
2. _____
3. _____

6/51
* make the commitment, join a group such as TOPS
* keep a diary
* establish realistic goals
* develop techniques to avoid overeating
* monitor your progress
* set a danger range at 3 or 4 pounds above your desired weight - don't let your weight exceed this amount.

Weight Management
Page #141

Identify four strategies for safe, effective weight loss.
1. _____
2. _____
3. _____
4. _____

Essay

6/52 Given the risks associated with dieting, how do you explain the huge commercial success enjoyed by manufacturers of diet products and authors of books on dieting?

6/53 Slimness has not always been the standard of beauty. Many cultures have different ideas about what is attractive. How do you think slimness came to be equated with beauty in America, and how is this image perpetuated?

6/54   Do you think that diet aids should be required to have written
        warnings on their labels regarding possible health risks? Why, or why
        not?

6/55   Do you think that weight loss programs that involve membership and
        participation in a group are more effective than individual weight
        management programs? What are the relative strengths and weaknesses
        of each?

Section II - Your Body: A Lifetime of Wellness

Chapter 7: Fitness

In this chapter -

* Lifelong Fitness
* Cardiovascular Fitness
* Muscular Strength
* Benefits of Exercise
* Exercise and Gender
* Nutrition
* Safety

Section II - Your Body: A Lifetime of Wellness
Chapter 7: Fitness

True-False

7/1   False
        Lifelong Fitness
        Page #146

The role of exercise in increasing the quality and length of life is not significant.

7/2   True
        Lifelong Fitness
        Page #146

A physically fit person can meet routine physical demands as well as unexpected challenges.

7/3   True
        Lifelong Fitness
        Page #147

Fitness is on the decline among young people in America.

7/4   False
        Cardiovascular Fitness
        Page #147

Anaerobic exercise boosts the body's consumption of oxygen.

7/5   True
        Cardiovascular Fitness
        Page #149

The most accurate measure of your level of exertion during exercise is your pulse, or heart rate.

7/6   True
        Cardiovascular Fitness
        Page #152

The physical benefits of exercise begin to fall off after a certain number of workouts each week.

7/7   False
        Cardiovascular Fitness
        Page #153

Jogging is America's most popular form of exercise.

7/8   False
        Muscular Strength
        Page #156

Aerobic exercise is an effective method of developing upper body muscle strength.

7/9   True
        Muscular Strength
        Page #157

Unused muscles will atrophy.

7/10   True
        Benefits of Exercise
        Page #161

Each hour of regular exercise adds 2 hours to your life.

7/11   False
        Benefits of Exercise
        Page #162

During exercise, your risk of heart attack is actually lower than when you are resting.

7/12   True
        Benefits of Exercise
        Page #163

Exercise may stop or prevent weak and brittle bones.

7/13   True   Men and women have similar responses to
Exercise and Gender   aerobic conditioning.
Page #164

7/14   False   Heavy exercise workouts increase your
Nutrition   body's need for protein.
Page #165

7/15   False   Safe exercise does not require special
Safety   equipment or clothing.
Pages #167-169

Mulitple Choice

7/16   a   The three components of fitness are
Lifelong Fitness   muscular strength and endurance,
Page #146   cardiovascular fitness, and

                                            a. flexibility.
                                            b. stamina.
                                            c. mental attitude.
                                            d. coordination.

7/17   b   The percentage of adult Americans who
Lifelong Fitness   report exercising regularly is
Page #148

                                            a. 59 percent.
                                            b. 69 percent.
                                            c. 79 percent.
                                            d. 89 percent.

7/18   d   The safest way to stretch is
Lifelong Fitness
Page #149   a. before your body temperature and
                                                muscles warm up.
                                            b. to push yourself just beyond your
                                                normal range of motion.
                                            c. with ballistic stretching.
                                            d. with static, or passive stretching.

7/19   c   Your target heart rate is equal to what
Cardiovascular Fitness   percentage of your maximum heart rate?
Page #151

                                            a. 80-85%
                                            b. 75-95%
                                            c. 65-85%
                                            d. 55-75%

7/20   a
Cardiovascular Fitness
Page #151

How long must you work out at your tar-get heart rate in order produce real benefits for your heart?

a. 15-20 minutes
b. 10-15 minutes
c. 5-10 minutes
d. 3-5 minutes

7/21   d
Cardiovascular Fitness
Page #152

What is the minimum number of workouts per week recommended by the American College of Sports Medicine?

a. 6
b. 5
c. 4
d. 3

7/22   c
Cardiovascular Fitness
Pages #152-153

Martin decides to take up walking in order to improve his level of cardio-vascular fitness. What combination of workout frequency (times per week) and workout length (minutes per workout) will safely provide aerobic benefits for Martin?

a. 2 workouts per week, 45 minutes each
b. 5 workouts per week, 45 minutes each
c. 3 workouts per week, 30 minutes each
d. 2 workouts per week, 15 minutes each

7/23   b
Cardiovascular Fitness
Page #154

Which of the following statements is the safest advice for someone who is considering taking up jogging?

a. Begin with repeated hard runs over a certain distance, followed by intervals of relaxed jogging.
b. Start by walking for 15 or 20 minutes, 3 times a week.
c. Begin by jogging for 10 minutes, and increase your time 1 or 2 minutes with each workout.
d. Wait at least three days after your first jog to run again.

7/24   b
Muscular Strength
Page #156

Which of the following is not the re-sult of exercising your muscles?

a. toughened muscle sheath
b. increased flexibility
c. improved circulation
d. increased amounts of connective tissue

7/25   d
        Muscular Strength
        Page #157

Exercises that provide overload resistance throughout the entire range of
motion are called

a. isometric
b. isotonic
c. isomorphic
d. isokinetic

7/26   c
        Muscular Strength
        Page #160

Regardless of which equipment you use
or which type of training you choose,
your muscles will not gain in strength
unless they are

a. stretched past the normal range of
   motion.
b. pushed to the "burn" point every 24
   hours.
c. overloaded so muscle failure occurs
   between 8 and 12 repetitions.
d. rested for at least 72 hours between
   workouts.

7/27   a
        Muscular Strength
        Page #161

Which of the following statements about
steroids is most accurate?

a. Steroids don't give athletes or
   body builders a competetive edge.
b. Steroids have adverse health effects
   for men, but not women.
c. Steroids have adverse health effects
   for women, but not men.
d. The illegitimate use of steroids is
   confined to adult athletes.

7/28   c
        Benefits of Exercise
        Page #162

Exercise contributes to increased
levels of high-density lipoproteins
(HDL) in the blood, thus reducing the
risk of

a. fibrinolysis.
b. osteoporosis.
c. coronary artery disease.
d. diabetes.

7/29   a
        Benefits of Exercise
        Page #163

Benefits of regular exercise include
mood elevation, protection from certain
cancers, stronger bones, and

a. lower weight.
b. reduced fibrinolosis.
c. elevated cholesterol levels.
d. reduced levels of endorphins.

7/30   b
Exercise and Gender
Page #164

Generally, women in training will lag behind men in

a. relative leg strength.
b. upper body strength.
c. reaction time.
d. amount of body fat.

7/31   d
Exercise and Gender
Page #164

Which of the following statements about men, women, and exercise is most accurate?

a. Men and women respond to aerobic conditioning differently.
b. Men and women have the same percentage of muscle mass to body weight.
c. A man and woman running at the same speed are working at the same levels of aerobic capacity.
d. In many fitness categories, there are greater differences between individuals of the same sex than between men and women.

7/32   b
Nutrition
Page #165

Glycogen, which is stored in the liver and acts as your body's fuel reserve during physical exertion, can be obtained most effectively by consuming

a. protein.
b. complex carbohydrates.
c. vitamins.
d. sucrose.

7/33   c
Nutrition
Page #166

Which of the following statements about exercise and nutrition is most accurate?

a. Carbohydrate loading has been proven to be a safe method of training.
b. Foods high in sugar content provide a sustained rush of energy.
c. As you sweat, the concentration of sodium in your blood actually increases.
d. Salt and electrolyte solutions are necessary after heavy sweating.

7/34   a
        Exercise and Rest
        Page #169

During sleep,

a. your body goes through a series of
   sleep stages about 4 or 5 times.
b. you dream most often during non-
   REM sleep stages.
c. brain activity remains fairly constant.
d. you spend most of your time dream-
   ing.

Matching

7/35   Directions: Match each of the temperature problems listed on the left
        with its correct description in the column on the right. Each
        description may be used only once.

Problem

1. __ Heat cramps
2. __ Heat stress
3. __ Heat exhaustion
4. __ Heat stroke
5. __ Frostnip
6. __ Frostbite
7. __ Hypothermia

Description

a. sudden blanching or lightening of
   the skin
b. excessive thirst, loss of coordination, increased sweating and
   body temperature
c. dry, hot skin; rapid pulse and
   breathing, coma or seizures
d. confusion, drowsiness, loss of
   coordination, coma
e. muscle twitching, cramping, or
   spasms
f. nausea, irritability, or vomiting
g. waxy looking skin with firm
   surface, pale appearance
h. fatigue, pale skin, low blood
   pressure, dizziness and blurred
   vision

1-e, 2-h, 3-b, 4-c,
5-a, 6-g, 7-h
Safety
Page #167

Completion

7/36
* find a partner
* choose an activity you genuinely enjoy
* set realistic goals
* find the best time of the day for a workout
* vary your routine
* monitor your progress
* commit yourself to a minimum of 8 weeks
Lifelong Fitness
Page #147

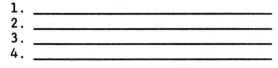

List four things you can do to get motivated to exercise.
1. _____
2. _____
3. _____
4. _____

7/37
If...
* you have, or have had, heart trouble/attack
* you feel pain/pressure in the left or mid-chest area, neck, shoulder or arm after exercising
* you often feel faint or have dizzy spells
* you are breathless after mild exertion
* you have high blood pressure that is not controlled
* you have bone or joint problems
* a member of your immediate family had a heart attack before the age of 50
* you have a medical condition that requires special attention
* you're over 40
Lifelong Fitness
Page #148

Identify 5 reasons to seek medical advice prior to starting an exercise
1. _____
2. _____
3. _____
4. _____
5. _____

7/38
* warm up for 5 minutes
* stretch for 5-10 minutes
* exercise at your target rate for at least 20 minutes 3 times per week
* cool down for 5 minutes by moving slowly
* stretch to prevent soreness the day after - about 5-10 minutes
Cardiovascular Fitness
Page #152

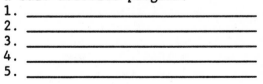

Identify the five basic steps of a safe aerobics program.
1. _____
2. _____
3. _____
4. _____
5. _____

7/39   * resting heart rate
Cardiovascular Fitness
Page #151

Michele has been sitting quietly for about 10 minutes, and finds her pulse to be beating 65 beats per minute. What is this rate called?

_____

7/40   * 120-157
Cardiovascular Fitness
Page #151

Lim is 35 years old, and has a maximum heart rate of 220 beats per minute. What is the <u>range</u> of his target heart rate?

beats per minute

_____

7/41   Sidestroke
Cardiovascular Fitness
Page #155

Which swimming stroke does <u>not</u> provide sufficient exertion to be of aerobic benefit?

_____

7/42   * warm up for 10 minutes
using static stretches
* never stretch past the
point of comfort
* wear proper shoes
* keep one foot on the
floor at all times
* stay low with knees bent
when moving side to side
Cardiovascular Fitness
Page #157

Identify four ways to "soften" your aerobic workout.
1. _____
2. _____
3. _____
4. _____

7/43   * don't train alone
* always warm up and stretch
before training
* begin with light weights,
and increase slowly until
the weight level causes
muscle failure anywhere
from 8-12 repetitions
* don't begin at maximum
level of exertion
* always use proper form
* always train your entire
body
* rest at least 48 hours, but
no more than 96 hours, between workouts
* quality performance is more
important than quantity
Muscular Strength
Page #160

A friend tells you that they are con-sidering taking up weight training, and asks your advice about how to go about it safely. List 5 safety tips.
1. _____
2. _____
3. _____
4. _____
5. _____

7/44
* increased risk of heart disease, stroke, or obstructed blood vessels
* increased aggression
* liver tumors and jaundice
* stunting of growth in adolescents
* acne
* risk of AIDS transmission if needles are used for injection and shared

Muscular Strength
Page #161

Your friends (male and female) in a local health club are talking about the benefits of anabolic steroids. What are three negative side effects or health risks associated with the use of steroids?
1. _____
2. _____
3. _____

7/45
* high-density lipoproteins (HDL)

Benefits
Page #161

Exercise benefits the heart and circulatory system by increasing blood levels of _____.

7/46
* Is it convenient/close by?
* What are the hours?
* Is it crowded during the times you will be there?
* Can you "try it out" before joining?
* Does it have complete facilities?
* What does membership include?
* Is long-term membership required?
* Are the trainers qualified?
* Do you like the atmosphere?

Benefits
Page #164

Identify five things to learn when considering joining a health club.
1. _____
2. _____
3. _____
4. _____
5. _____

7/47
* replace fluids lost through sweat with water
* don't rely on thirst as an indicator of water need
* drink small amounts of cool water (5-6 oz) at 15 minute intervals during vigorous exercise
* drink 2-4 cups cold water about 10 minutes before a race, 1-2 cups during the race
* for each pound lost during workouts, drink one half quart of water; monitor your weight loss after training

Nutrition
Page #166

State three ways to prevent dehydration.
1. _____
2. _____
3. _____

7/48   * keep regular hours for
       going to bed and getting
       up in the morning
       * exercise every day
       * don't drink coffee in the
       evening
       * don't smoke
       * don't use alcohol to get
       to sleep
       * don't nap during the day
       * don't go to bed starved or
       stuffed
       * develop a sleep ritual
       * get a good mattress
       Rest
       Page #169

List five things you can do to improve
your sleeping habits.
1. _____
2. _____
3. _____
4. _____
5. _____

7/49   * choose an activity you
       genuinely enjoy
       * start slowly and proceed
       gradually
       * don't overwork your body
       * stop and take stock of
       your progress regularly
       * schedule your activity
       into your life - get it on
       your calendar
       Lifelong Fitness
       Page #170

Your friend wants to begin an exercise
program. Give three suggestions for
helping her get off to a good start.
1. _____
2. _____
3. _____

Essay

7/50   How do you explain America's fascination with fitness? Specifical-
       ly, do Americans really want to be fit, do they just want to look
       good, or both?

7/51   If you're involved in an exercise program, discuss your reasons for
       getting/staying involved. If you're not, try to describe why you
       haven't made the choice to get in shape. How are you different from
       others you know who are exercising regularly? Are your reasons valid?

7/52   Increasing numbers of women are taking up body building and weight
       training. What do you think motivates these women to develop their
       muscular strength and appearance? Are they the same reasons that
       motivate men to become involved in weight training?

7/53   The food supplement industry is now heavily involved in the fitness
       movement with protein pills, vitamin supplements, and weight control
       products. Do you think this industry needs regulation in order to
       protect the health of its consumers? Why, or why not?

7/54   America seems to have turned its back on children when it comes to
       fitness. Why do you suppose the fitness movement hasn't made more
       inroads into the public education system of our country?

7/55   Describe the level of fitness necessary for maximum enjoyment of your present lifestyle. How does your present level of fitness compare? What changes, if any, do you think are necessary?

<u>AN INVITATION TO HEALTH</u>
TEST BANK

Section II - Your Body: A Lifetime of Wellness

<u>Chapter 8: Aging</u>

In this chapter -

*   Aging Process
*   Successful Aging
*   Problems
*   Extending Life
*   Aging Society

Section II - Your Body: A Lifetime of Wellness
Chapter 8: Aging

True-False

8/1	True Aging Process Page #174	The historical view of aging as simply a process of deterioration into frailty and dementia is no longer considered valid.
8/2	False Aging Process Page #174	All aging changes and patterns begin at birth.
8/3	False Aging Process Page #176	The effects of physical decline in the body become obvious around the age of 30.
8/4	True Successful Aging Page #177	Many of the losses linked to age are the result of a sedentary lifestyle.
8/5	False Successful Aging Page #178	Aging is now viewed as a single process that invariably causes progressive decline.
8/6	True Successful Aging Page #178	Intellectual ability does not necessarily decline along with physical vigor.
8/7	True Problems Page #183	Osteoporosis is most effectively prevented by insuring adequate calcium intake during adolescence.
8/8	True Problems Page #182	According to recent surveys, Americans under the age of 65 tend to overestimate the seriousness of problems for the elderly such as poverty and loneliness.
8/9	False Problems Page #184	The elderly are at low risk for the abuse or misuse of drugs.
8/10	False Problems Page #184	Half of the Americans over the age of 65 live in nursing homes.
8/11	True Extending Life Page #187	Other than the giant tortoise, only humans live to be over 100 years of age.

Chapter 8: Aging

8/12   True
    Extending Life
    Page #187

Most nutritional approaches to extending life have not been validated in tests with humans.

8/13   False
    Extending Life
    Page #187

Between 1900 and 1980, the percentage of the population living to age 85 has increased.

8/14   True
    Extending Life
    Page #188

Loss of ability to moderate the stress response is believed to be associated with the aging process.

8/15   True
    Aging Society
    Page #190

By the year 2000, the median age in America will be 35 years.

Multiple Choice

8/16   b
    Aging Process
    Page #174

The key to staying healthy and vital in old age is

a. supplementing your diet with vitamins.
b. maintaining healthful behaviors throughout life.
c. exercising regularly after the age of 50.
d. minimizing physical activity after the age of 30.

8/17   a
    Aging Process
    Page #175

Which of the following statements about middle age is most accurate?

a. For women, middle age seems to be a time of increasing happiness.
b. For men, middle age is a time of emotional stability and well-being.
c. Physical changes are more profound for men than women during middle age.
d. Menopause occurs over a period of about 20 years.

8/18   d
    Aging Process
    Page #176

Which of the following is not a change associated with the aging process?

a. gradual decrease in the heart's ability to pump blood
b. lowering of the basal metabolism
c. loss of height
d. decline in intelligence

8/19   c
        Successful Aging
        Page #177

Research into the role of heredity and aging shows that

a. the rate of aging is predetermined by heredity.
b. inactivity slows the aging process.
c. exercise slows the aging process.
d. twins live longer than normal.

8/20   a
        Successful Aging
        Page #177

The aging process affects the brain

a. by slowing the process of cell repair and replacement.
b. by preventing self-repair of the brain during Alzheimer's disease.
c. by causing irreversible declines in intelligence.
d. in a simple process of progressive decline.

8/21   b
        Successful Aging
        Page #179

Which of the following is not a mental problem for people over the age of 60?

a. naming and language retrieval
b. compensating for memory loss
c. organizing new information
d. distractions and lack of focus

8/22   c
        Problems
        Page #182

Osteoporosis is a significant health risk for older adults

a. because of the expense of calcium supplements.
b. only if they are Asian or White female.
c. because of the increased chance of fracture.
d. unless they drank milk during adolescence.

8/23   d
        Problems
        Page #184

The most commonly misused drugs among the elderly are sleeping pills, pain medication, tranquilizers, and

a. amphetamines.
b. antacids.
c. vitamin supplements.
d. laxatives.

8/24   d
        Problems
        Page #184

The number of Americans over the age of 65 who fall below the poverty line is

a. 0.5 million.
b. 1.5 million.
c. 2.5 million.
d. 3.5 million.

8/25   c
        Problems
        Page #185

Assisting older adults with daily living activities

a. is usually limited to those in poor health.
b. is rarely done by other older adults.
c. is frequently done by other older adults.
d. is becoming easier because of the increasing number of elderly who live with their children's families.

8/26   b
        Problems
        Page #186

Alzheimer's disease

a. is a form of mental illness.
b. presents symptoms similar to many other unrelated conditions.
c. is characterized by the abnormal production of brain cells.
d. can be cured if detected early.

8/27   a
        Extending Life
        Page #187

Human longevity may be determined by the phenomenon called limited cell doubling, that limits the number of times body cells may double to about

a. 50.
b. 75.
c. 100.
d. 150.

8/28   c
        Aging Society
        Page #190

Which of the following is not likely to be a consequence of a "graying" America?

a. changes in the Social Security system
b. increase in funding for programs for the elderly
c. continuation of present policies that determine how health care costs are distributed
d. increased elderly involvement in higher education

8/29   b
Aging Process
Page #175

Physical changes for men during middle age include prostate gland changes and a slowing of sexual response caused by

a. increased testosterone levels.
b. decreased testosterone levels.
c. the climacteric.
d. a decrease in the level of estrogen.

8/30   d
Successful Aging
Page #181

Which of the following statements about aging and mental health is most accurate?

a. Good mental and emotional health is not related to the rate of aging.
b. The elderly are more vulnerable to mental illness.
c. The prevalence of clinical depression is higher during old age than at earlier stages of development.
d. Death rates are higher for older adults without strong social ties.

8/31   a
Successful Aging
Page #181

Research reports that the sexual response of postmenopausal women

a. increased or remained the same for 80% of those surveyed.
b. decreased for 80% of those surveyed.
c. was unchanged for 20% of those surveyed.
d. was characterized by a decline in sexual pleasure.

8/32

a
Successful Aging
Pages #181-182

The most important thing you can do to insure a successful retirement is

a. plan your new routine.
b. concentrate totally on saving enough money.
c. relax, and do as little as necessary.
d. let your spouse manage his/her retirement on their own.

8/33   d
Problems
Page #182

Factors contributing to osteoporosis include declining bone mass caused by aging and falling levels of hormones (in women), inadequate calcium, and

a. genetic traits.
b. number of bone fractures.
c. body weight.
d. cigarette smoking or alcohol intake.

8/34   b
        Problems
        Page #183

Effective treatments for osteoporosis include estrogen and

a. increased caffeine intake.
b. exercise.
c. avoidance of sunlight.
d. vitamin A supplements.

8/35   c
        Problems
        Page #185

The likelihood of living alone rises most dramatically

a. for men under 65 years.
b. for men over 65 years.
c. for women generally as they grow older.
d. for women over 85 years.

Completion

8/36   * watch your weight
        * eat a low-fat, balanced diet
        * don't smoke
        * get regular medical exams
        * keep high blood pressure under control
        * avoid anti-aging gimmicks
        * try to avoid accidents
        * balance your work and play
        * exercise regularly
        Aging Process
        Page #174

Now that you've read the chapter on aging, you're considering what to do in order to live longer. List five tips for staying younger longer.

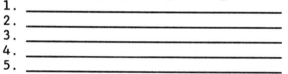

1. _____
2. _____
3. _____
4. _____
5. _____

8/37   * relaxation of roles
        * greater assertiveness in women
        * greater expressiveness in men
        * freedom to pick up and go
        * more time for yourself
        * greater tolerance for others
        * more companionship with your mate
        * new relationship with children
        * opportunity to make contributions to community, history, or culture
        Aging Process
        Page #175

Your best friend has just turned 50, and is complaining about how "life is just about over." Identify five new potentials or special strengths common to people between 45 and 60 years of age.

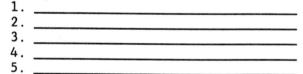

1. _____
2. _____
3. _____
4. _____
5. _____

8/38
* get a checkup before starting an exercise program
* warm up and stretch properly before exercising
* try walking for aerobic training
* avoid quick movements or situations in which you're likely to fall
* build unprogrammed exercise into your daily schedule
Successful Aging
Page #177

List three tips for staying fit after the age of 50.
1. _____
2. _____
3. _____

8/39
* 1,500 mg per day
Problems
Page #183

Your friend Moira went through menopause about a year ago, and is concerned about her calcium intake. What is the recommended daily amount of calcium for postmenopausal women?
_____

8/40
* get regular, but not excessive, exercise
* reduce caffeine intake, drink coffee with skim milk
* drink only moderate amounts of alcohol
* don't smoke
* get enough vitamin D
* investigate estrogen supplements if you've been through menopause
Problems
Page #183

List four things you can do, other than monitor your calcium intake, to prevent osteoporosis.
1. _____
2. _____
3. _____
4. _____

8/41
* a female, aged 75 or older, who is dependent upon the abuser for food and shelter
Problems
Page #187

Describe the average victim of elder abuse.
_____
_____
_____

8/42
* declining organ reserve
Extending Life
Page #187

The functional capacity of the heart, lungs, kidney, and liver begins to decline around age 30, and may determine longevity. What is this theory called?
_____

8/43
* do nothing in excess
* get up early
* have faith in a higher power
* keep busy
* be self-sufficient and self-protective
Extending Life
Page #189

What can you do to live to be 100 years old? List four strategies.
1. _____
2. _____
3. _____
4. _____

8/44
* heredity (+/-)
* smoking (-)
* alcohol in moderation(+)
* heavy alcohol intake (-)
* poor diet (-)
* excess body weight (-)
* appropriate exercise (+)
* reduced stress (+)
* interest/involvement in life (+)
Aging Society
Page #190

There are a number of variables that influence lifespan. List 6, and indicate whether they increase (+) or decrease (-) your lifespan.
1. _____ ( )
2. _____ ( )
3. _____ ( )
4. _____ ( )
5. _____ ( )
6. _____ ( )

Essay

8/45   Discuss the relationship between the high value our society places on independence and the dilemma of older adults who must depend on others for assistance with daily activities. Specifically, how does our value system affect our expectations for the elderly, and their caretakers?

8/46   Putting older adults "out to pasture" is a waste of human potential and resources. What unique contributions do you think older adults can make to their communities? Why aren't these opportunities explored more aggressively?

8/47   Growing old in a society that values youth can be difficult and painful. What would you recommend an older adult do to prevent feeling worthless and unappreciated?

8/48   What role should state, local, and national government agencies play in assisting the elderly? Specifically, what kind of programs for older adults would you be willing to support with your tax dollars?

8/49   How long do you think you're going to live? Why?

8/50   If you had to choose between saving the life of an older adult or a young child, who would you save? At what point would their relative ages no longer be a factor?

AN INVITATION TO HEALTH
TEST BANK

Section III - Your Sexuality: Responsibility
and Rewards

Chapter 9: Intimate Relationships

In this chapter -

*   Relationships
*   Marriage

AN INVITATION TO HEALTH
Test Bank

Section III - Your Sexuality: Responsibility
and Rewards
Chapter 9: Intimate Relationships

True-False

9/1	True Relationships Page #197	Interpersonal relationships are essential to human life.
9/2	False Relationships Page #197	Intimacy means having a sexual relationship with another person.
9/3	True Relationships Page #197	Our relationships with other people are based on the way we perceive ourselves.
9/4	False Relationships Page #199	The components of friendship (respect, loyalty, and tolerance) are valued only in Western cultures.
9/5	False Relationships Page #200	The primary purpose of dating is to establish a sexual relationship with another person.
9/6	True Relationships Page #202	In an intimate and mature loving relationship, each partner's problems, goals, and identity remain separate.
9/7	True Marriage Page #202	Traditionally, marriages were arranged for economic or political reasons.
9/8	False Marriage Page #202	The divorce rate is rising.
9/10	True Marriage Page #202	Marriages between people under the age of 20 are at increased risk of failure.
9/11	True Marriage Page #202	Mature love is defined by experts on marriage as caring as much about another's happiness and needs as your own.
9/12	False Marriage Page #202	The best indicators of success for a marriage are the religious backgrounds of the bride and groom.

9/13   True
            Marriage
            Page #204

The majority of families with children under age 18 are headed by two-career couples.

9/14   False
            Marriage
            Page #205

While marriage may make people happier, there is no difference in the physical health status of married and unmarried adults.

9/15   True
            Marriage
            Page #210

Reported rates of marital satisfaction tend to fall slightly after the birth of the first child.

9/16   True
            Marriage
            Page #212

Marital therapy has been shown to be an effective method for improving relationships.

Multiple Choice

9/17   d
            Relationships
            Page #198

In order to develop intimacy, one must have the capacity to

a. exist in relationships without the need for help or support.
b. maintain regular sexual activity.
c. be brutally honest.
d. share close, confidential communi-cation.

9/18   c
            Relationships
            Page #199

Which of the following statements about friendship is most accurate?

a. Deep and lasting friendships are quite common.
b. Friendships between men are based on factors different than friendships between women.
c. Friendship plays some of the roles traditionally performed by extended families.
d. Friendships formed during adolesence are usually shallow and temporary.

9/19   a
       Relationships
       Page #200

The first step in making responsible
sexual decisions is

a. understanding and respecting the
   sexual values of yourself and your
   partner.
b. obtaining the proper form of birth
   control.
c. to start fresh; don't be concerned
   about your partner's previous experiences.
d. to remember that sex is supposed to
   be awkward and a little intimidating.

9/20   b
       Relationships
       Page #200

One important difference between lasting love and infatuation is that

a. infatuation rarely involves sexual
   feelings.
b. love lasts, and infatuation doesn't.
c. love can be a disguise for something
   quite different like fear of loneli-
   ness.
d. love evokes serious feelings, and
   infatuation doesn't.

9/21   b
       Marriage
       Page #202

Which of the following is not an advantage of arranged marriages?

a. The partners are more likely to have
   similar values.
b. The couple's relationship is more
   intimate than with conventional
   marriage arrangements.
c. They are an effective tool for dealing with the stress of living in a
   foreign country.
d. They promote cultural and religious
   continuity.

9/22   c
       Marriage
       Page #202

Pragmatic reasons for marrying include

a. physical and sexual drives.
b. the pleasure and satisfaction of
   love.
c. pregnancy and escape from authority.
d. innate dependency needs.

9/23   a
       Marriage
       Page #203

We tend to marry people from similar
social backgrounds and the same

a. geographical area we grew up in.
b. lifestyle as our parent's had.
c. values regarding money and finance.
d. astrological sign.

9/24   d
        Marriage
        Page #204

An egalitarian marriage is one in which

a. both partners work.
b. each partner is responsible for 50% of the assets.
c. the roles of fathering and mothering are secondary to the rewards of partnership.
d. all aspects of life are shared equally.

9/25   c
        Marriage
        Pages #204-205

Working wives and mothers frequently

a. sacrifice some of their health and happiness in order to make ends meet.
b. get a job for reasons other than financial need.
c. are more stressed than women who don't work outside the home.
d. quit soon after starting their job.

9/26   b
        Marriage
        Page #205

Which of the following statements regarding marriage and health is most accurate?

a. Married men are more prone to alcoholism than their unmarried peers.
b. Separation and divorce have been linked to drops in immune function.
c. A single person is just as likely to be happy and satisfied with life as a married person.
d. Single women live longer than married women.

9/27   a
        Marriage
        Page #210

Married couples should have intercourse

a. that is mutually satisfying, and not worry about what the "average" couple is doing.
b. at least 3 times per week.
c. at the same frequency as when they were first married.
d. enough times each week to satisfy the more sexually active partner.

9/28   d
        Marriage
        Page #211

A spouse's response to infidelity by by their partner usually includes feeling betrayed, denial, guilt, anger or depression, and ultimately

a. divorce.
b. suicide.
c. an extramarital affair of their own.
d. a rekindled sense of competency.

9/29
c
Marriage
Page #211

Unexpressed feelings and unrealistic expectations can cause trouble for a marriage unless they are communicated without blame, real causes of anger are identified, and

a. each partner generalizes their feelings of resentment.
b. feelings of resentment are expressed at every opportunity.
c. each partner is willing to change.
d. the partner at fault is willing to change.

9/30
a
Marriage
Page #214

Which of the following statements about divorce is most accurate?

a. The remarriage rate increases with the number of times a person is divorced.
b. The remarriage rate decreases with the number of divorces.
c. The divorce rate has climbed steadily throughout the eighties.
d. 60% of all marriages now end in divorce.

9/31
b
Alternatives
Page #214

Living together (but not married) means

a. avoiding many of the interpersonal problems associated with marriage.
b. doing without certain legal rights provided to married couples.
c. less stressful relationships with parents and relatives.
d. settling for a less satisfying relationship.

Completion

9/32
* know your own feelings
* use eye contact
* consider both points of view
* paraphrase what your partner is saying if you don't understand
* make positive statements
* be specific about your wants and desires
* don't expect your partner to be a mind reader
* listen when you're finished talking
Relationships
Page #198

Identify five ways to develop effective interpersonal communication.

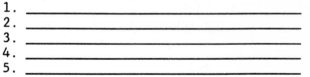

1. _____
2. _____
3. _____
4. _____
5. _____

9/33

* be willing to open up
* be sensitive to his
  friend's feelings
* express appreciation
* see his friends clearly;
  it's OK to recognize
  faults
* enjoy during the good
  times, stay involved dur-
  difficulties
* expect occasional disap-
  pointment
* talk about the friendship
Relationships
Page #199

Your friend Bert has expressed a desire
to improve his relationships with other
people. List four things Bert can do
to develop and maintain closeness with
his friends.

1. _____
2. _____
3. _____
4. _____

9/34

* recognize and act on her
  values regarding sex
* communicate her feelings
  when she feels pressured
* avoid acting or talking
  suggestively
* think ahead to avoid
  letting unanticipated
  events dictate what
  happens
* speak up early about what
  she wants to happen
* not to give in to emo-
  tional blackmail
* not to be afraid to end
  a relationship that is
  based exclusively on sex
Relationships
Page #200

The daughter of a friend has approached
you because she feels pressured to have
sex when out on a date. Identify four
things she could do if she's not interested in having sex.

1. _____
2. _____
3. _____
4. _____

9/35

* you don't feel comfort-
  able when you're together
* you feel angry or letdown
  after being together
* your partner is secretive
  about his/her life
* your partner isn't atten-
  tive to you
* you don't feel cared for
  or appreciated
Relationships
Page #201

You have been dating someone for some
time now, but aren't sure whether or
not to continue. Identify three criteria that would indicate its time to
end the relationship.

1. _____
2. _____
3. _____

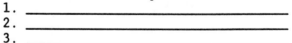

9/36
* neither of you are sure of the other's love
* most of your time together is spent quarreling
* you're both under age 20
* you think your partner will change after marriage
* your partner has traits or behaviors that truly bother you
* your partner wants you to make changes that will limit your satisfaction with your life
Marriage
Page #203

Give four reasons for <u>not</u> getting married.
1. _____
2. _____
3. _____
4. _____

9/37
* commitment
Marriage
Page #204

Shared values, willingness to tolerate flaws and be responsive, a match in religious beliefs, and good communication skills are all crucial compatibilities for _____.

9/38
* plan your weekends
* keep dating
* spend regular time alone together
* be supportive with each other
* accept and give help
Marriage
Page #205

You and your spouse both have full-time jobs for the first time in your married life. Identify three things you can do to keep the stress level manageable.
1. _____
2. _____
3. _____

9/39
* talk about how you feel; use "I," not "you"
* be clear about the issue
* don't embarrass each other or be intimidating
* avoid generalizations
* be fair and honest
* focus on the present
* think before talking
* learn to listen
* don't force agreement
Marriage
Page #209

Name five guidelines for fighting fairly.
1. _____
2. _____
3. _____
4. _____
5. _____

9/40
* be informed and set realistic expectations
* expect and express your negative feelings
* take time for you and your spouse
* talk with other parents
* focus on the positives
Marriage
Page #210

Having a child can be stressful for a couple. Name three strategies for dealing with the changes brought about by parenthood.
1. _____
2. _____
3. _____

9/41
* personal bias of the
  author
* faulty methodology
Marriage
Page #213

Recent research by "cultural historian" Shere Hite revealed a discouraging picture of marriage in America. In spite of its popularity, her work was found to have two basic flaws. What are they?
1. _____
2. _____

9/42
* focus on your spouse's
  positive qualities
* learn to negotiate
* look behind surface problems
* keep your perspective
* focus on opportunities for
  improvement
Marriage
Page #212

List three tips for staying married.
1. _____
2. _____
3. _____

9/43
* fill your life with meaningful work and people
* build a social support
  network
* be open to new experiences
* don't miss out on a special event just because
  you have to go alone
* volunteer your time and
  energy to those less for-
  tunate
Alternatives
Page #214

Living alone doesn't have to be lonely. Name four things you can do to keep living alone from becoming lonely.
1. _____
2. _____
3. _____
4. _____

9/44
* inquire about your partner's feelings, interests,
  and thoughts
* treat your partner as a
  complete person
* work as a team
* spend some time each day
  focusing exclusively on
  your partner
* develop common interests
* learn to be a better lover
* don't play games
* be polite
* give as much of yourself
  as you can
Relationships
Page #215

List five ways to make a relationship more meaningful.
1. _____
2. _____
3. _____
4. _____
5. _____

Matching

9/45   Directions: Match each of the marriage styles on the left with its
        correct definition on the right. Each definition may be used only
        once.

	Style		Definition
1.	__ traditional		a. partners are together for prag-
2.	__ companion-oriented		matic reasons
3.	__ utilitarian		b. the rewards of partnerships are
4.	__ egalitarian		the primary basis for marriage
5.	__ androgynous		c. the relationship is primarily a

Style
1.   __ traditional
2.   __ companion-oriented
3.   __ utilitarian
4.   __ egalitarian
5.   __ androgynous

Definition
a. partners are together for pragmatic reasons
b. the rewards of partnerships are
   the primary basis for marriage
c. the relationship is primarily a
   financial one
d. couples take on culturally prescribed roles
e. all apects of life are divided
   equally
f. neither partner is bound to traditional roles

1-d, 2-b, 3-a, 4-e, 5-f
Marriage
Page #204

Essay

9/46   Discuss some of the ways that we learn about relationships from our
        parents. Specifically, how does the way they conduct their marriage
        affect the way we view commitment and intimacy?

9/47   Historically, marriages were arranged for economic reasons. Consider
        the following statement, and then present a brief argument (either
        agreeing or disagreeing) with evidence to support your views.

        "Marriage in contemporary American society has even greater economic
        significance than it did 100 years ago."

9/48   What are your personal criteria for a successful relationship?
        Develop a brief list of factors you consider important and support
        your choices with examples or experiences you've had.

9/49   Divorce has profound and often tragic consequences for the children
        involved. Provide a brief critique of the following proposal to
        reduce the damage caused by divorce.

        Marriage, as we know it, should be deregulated entirely. Couples
        should be allowed to do whatever they want together **except have
        children**. The right to bear and raise children should be determined
        by some formal process of evaluation. Couples interested in having
        children should be required to obtain a license based on their ability
        to parent and nuture children. Children should only be born to
        parents willing and able to care for them adequately. Society can't
        afford the cost of divorces that involve children.

Chapter 9: Intimate Relationships

9/50   This chapter has discussed several types of marriage (egalitarian, utilitarian, etc.). Are there also different types of friendship? If so, what are they? If not, why not?

<u>AN INVITATION TO HEALTH</u>
TEST BANK

Section III - Your Sexuality: Responsibility
and Rewards

<u>Chapter 10: Sexuality</u>

In this chapter -

*   Gender Identity
*   Sexual Development
*   Sexual Preference
*   Sexual Behavior
*   Sexual Response
*   Sexual Problems
*   Victims

Section III - Your Sexuality: Responsibility
and Rewards
Chapter 10: Sexuality

True-False

10/1	False Gender Identity Page #219	The term sexuality refers to the stages of physical arousal you experience during sexual activity.
10/2	True Gender Identity Page #219	Your gender identity is molded through the process of socialization.
10/3	True Gender Identity Page #220	Sexual stereotyping results in diminished quality of life for many women.
10/4	True Sexual Development Page #223	Sexual development is driven by the release of hormones.
10/5	False Sexual Development Page #223	Sexual development does not really begin until puberty.
10/6	False Sexual Development Page #224	Sexual development is complete by the time we reach adulthood.
10/7	True Sexual Preference Page #225	Our attraction to a certain sex is determined by physiological, social, and psychological factors.
10/8	False Sexual Preference Page #225	Homosexuality and heterosexuality represent separate and independent orientations to sexual attraction.
10/9	True Sexual Behavior Page #225	Understanding the diversity of sexual behavior is important in learning to accept our own sexual feelings.
10/10	True Sexual Behavior Page #228	Fantasy plays a positive role in the human sexual experience.
10/11	False Sexual Behavior Page #229	Heterosexual intercourse is the most common form of sexual activity.

10/12	False Sexual Response Page #231	The physical aspects of sexual response differ depending on the type of sexual stimulation taking place.
10/13	True Sexual Problems Page #233	Sexual difficulties may occur at any point during the sexual response sequence.
10/14	False Sexual Problems Page #234	Impotence is primarily a psychological problem.
10/15	True Victims Pages #238-239	The incidence of rape is increasing faster than any other violent crime in America.

Multiple Choice

10/16   a
Gender Identity
Page #219

Sex differences between men and women include bone size, hair growth, locations of fat deposits, and

a. earlier physical maturation for women.
b. earlier physical maturation for men.
c. longer life expectancy for men.
d. lower sensitivity to taste, heat and noise for women.

10/17   d
Gender Identity
Page #221

Sexual stereotyping

a. begins in adolescence.
b. is a recent phenomenon of American culture.
c. does not have a particularly strong impact on those affected by it.
d. equates being male with masculinity, and being female with femininity.

10/18   c
Gender Identity
Page #223

Which of the following statements about masculinity and femininity is most accurate?

a. Americans place a higher value on traits assigned as "feminine" over those seen as "masculine."
b. Gender identity and sex-role behavior are determined socially.
c. A man who stays home to care for his children is exhibiting androgynous behavior.
d. Sex roles are constant across different cultures.

10/19   b
Sexual Development
Page #223

Childhood sexuality

a. lasts from birth to age 6.
b. is characterized in part by curiosity about sex and reproduction.
c. involves the release of gonado-
   tropins.
d. begins with the recognition of
   genital differences between boys and
   girls.

10/20   b
Sexual Development
Page #223

Hormones affecting sexual development

a. are produced in the pituitary
   gland.
b. act on certain cells and organs to
   perform specific functions.
c. are identical for men and women.
d. are regulated by the gonads.

10/21   d
Sexual Development
Page #224

Which of the following is not an
accurate description of adolescent
sexuality?

a. It begins in the brain.
b. It is characterized by rapid
   physiological changes.
c. Curiosity about sex conflicts with
   established social and cultural
   values.
d. The menarche marks the end of
   sexual maturation for females.

10/22   a
Sexual Development
Page #224

The average age for first intercourse
is now less than

a. 15 years.
b. 16 years.
c. 17 years.
d. 18 years.

10/23   c
Sexual Preference
Page #226

Sexual orientation

a. remains constant throughout life.
b. is biologically determined.
c. in America is primarily hetero-
   sexual.
d. can be either exclusively homosexual
   or exclusively heterosexual.

10/24 c
Sexual Preference
Page #222

Which of the following statements about homosexuality is most accurate?

a. The presence of homosexuality is limited to industrialized societies.
b. Homosexual lifestyles are inherently more stressful than their hetero-sexual counterparts.
c. No single social or psychological cause of homosexuality has been identified.
d. One impact of the AIDS epidemic has been a lessening of homophobia.

10/25 a
Sexual Behavior
Page #228

Erotic fantasies

a. are a common form of enhancing sexual arousal.
b. are limited to those dissatisfied with their sex life.
c. are completely different depending on one's sexual orientation.
d. usually express socially acceptable forms of sexual behavior.

10/26 c
Sexual Behavior
Page #228

Which of the following forms of sexual activity is least likely to result in the transmission of disease?

a. cunnilingus
b. coitus
c. celibacy
d. fellatio

10/27 b
Sexual Behavior
Page #229

The best form of sexual activity

a. is the one that guarantees orgasm for everyone involved.
b. depends almost completely on the preferences, values, and needs of the people involved.
c. involves a partner of a different sex.
d. is against the law in many states.

10/28   c   William Masters and Virginia Johnson,
          Sexual Response   the pioneers of research in sexual
          Page #231   response, concluded that

                                a. men and women have distinctly dif-
                                   ferent patterns of sexual response.
                                b. sexual response is a well-ordered
                                   sequence of three basic events.
                                c. the physiology of sexual response is
                                   the same regardless of the method of
                                   stimulation.
                                d. real life sexual behavior always
                                   follows the same pattern.

10/29   a   Which of the following is _not_ one of
          Sexual Response   phases of sexual response identified
          Pages #231-232   by Masters and Johnson?

                                a. withdrawal
                                b. resolution
                                c. plateau
                                d. excitement

10/30   d   Orgasm
          Sexual Response
          Page #232   a. is virtually the same for men and
                                   women.
                                b. involves contractions for men, but
                                   not for women.
                                c. for women involves a single pattern
                                   consisting of a series of mini-
                                   organisms.
                                d. for men and women is differentiated
                                   primarily by the fact that men
                                   ejaculate, and women don't.

10/31   a   The length of the refractory period, or
          Sexual Response   time during which the man is incapable
          Page #232   of having another orgasm,

                                a. can be anywhere from several minutes
                                   to several days.
                                b. is not affected by previous sexual
                                   activity.
                                c. is determined by the man's age.
                                d. is usually equal to the amount of
                                   time engaged in intercourse.

10/32   b
         Sexual Problems
         Page #233

Which of the following statements about sexual difficulties is most accurate?

a. Sexual difficulties usually occur in the orgasm phase of sexual response.
b. The most frequent problem seen by sex therapists is lack of sexual desire.
c. Sexual problems are almost always psychological in nature.
d. A person who has never experienced orgasm may be said to have a secondary difficulty.

10/33   d
         Sexual Problems
         Pages #235-236

Which of the following is not a male sexual problem?

a. impotence
b. premature ejaculation
c. sexual anxiety
d. dyspareunia

10/34   c
         Sexual Response
         Pages #235-237

Problems in the orgasm phase of sexual response

a. appear most often for men in the form of impotence.
b. are limited primarily to women who can't achieve orgasm.
c. can be treated in a variety of ways.
d. occur for individuals regardless of whether they are masturbating or involved with a partner.

10/35   b
         Atypical Behavior
         Page #238

Characteristics exhibited by sexual addicts include using sex to hide from troubles, large amounts of time spent seeking partners, a compulsion to have repeated sex or engage in behavior that produces guilty feelings, and

a. high levels of sexual self-esteem.
b. a preoccupation with sex that interferes with an ongoing sexual relationship.
c. inability to achieve orgasm.
d. an overabundance of sex hormmones.

10/36   a
Victims
Page #239

Which of the following statements about rape is <u>not</u> accurate?

a. Only 30% of all rapes are planned.
b. Children, old women, nuns, and pregnant women are all at risk.
c. Most rapes are not reported to the police.
d. The effect of rape on the victim is devastating.

10/36   d
Victims
Page #242

Children who suffer sexual abuse

a. rarely know the abuser.
b. tend to blame their parents after the incident.
c. usually tell their parents about it right away.
d. often believe they have done something wrong.

10/37   c
Business
Page #242

Prostitution and pornography

a. are not significant problems from a financial standpoint.
b. are problems limited to modern societies.
c. present health, as well as social and moral, risks.
d. cause sexually violent crimes.

Matching

10/38   Directions: Match each part of the female sexual anatomy listed on
         the left with its correct description on the right. Each
         description may be used only once.

	Anatomical Name	Description
1.	__ mons pubis	a. the opening to the uterus, found at the back of the vagina
2.	__ labia majora	b. most sensitive spot in genital area
3.	__ labia minora	c. canal leading to primary internal reproductive organs
4.	__ clitoris	d. egg cell
5.	__ urethra	e. area between vagina and rectum
6.	__ vagina	f. hair-covered area over the pubic bone
7.	__ perineum	g. outer lips of female genitalia
8.	__ cervix	h. also called the womb
9.	__ uterus	i. inner lips of female genitalia
10.	__ fallopian tube	j. opening of tube to bladder
11.	__ ovary	k. canal from uterus to ovary
		l. site of female sex hormone production.

1-f, 2-g, 3-i, 4-b, 5-j,
6-c, 7-e, 8-a, 9-h, 10-k, 11-l
Gender Identity
Page #220

10/39   Directions: Match each part of the male sexual anatomy listed on the
         left with its correct description on the right. Each description
         may be used only once.

	Anatomical Name	Description
1.	__ penis	a. carries sperm from the testes
2.	__ scrotum	b. coiled tubes, site of sperm storage
3.	__ testes	c. secrete small amounts of fluid during arousal
4.	__ epididymis	d. pouch containing the testes
5.	__ vas deferens	e. seminal fluid
6.	__ prostate gland	f. combination of muscle, loose skin, and hollow cylinders
7.	__ semen	g. manufacture testosterone
8.	__ Cowper's glands	h. sperm cells
9.	__ seminal vesicles	i. where some seminal fluid is made
		j. liquid in which sperm are carried
		k. where sperm and seminal fluid are mixed

1-f, 2-d, 3-g, 4-b,
5-a, 6-k, 7-j, 8-c, 9-i
Gender Identity
Page #221

10/40   Directions: Match each of the sexual deviations on the left with its correct description on the right. Each description may be used only once.

Deviation

1. __ fetishism
2. __ pedophilia
3. __ transvestism
4. __ exhibitionism
5. __ voyeurism
6. __ sadism
7. __ masochism

Description

a. sexual arousal by inflicting pain
b. sexual gratification through observation of others involved in sex
c. sexual pleasure from object or a- sexual body part
d. sexual gratification by suffering physical or psychological pain
e. sexual pleasure through fantasy
f. sex between an adult and child
g. exhibiting one's genitals to an unwilling observer
h. sexual arousal by wearing clothes of opposite sex

1-c, 2-f, 3-h, 4-g,
5-b, 6-a, 7-d
Atypical Behavior
Page #238

Completion

10/41   * sexual stereotyping
         Gender Identity
         Page #221

Equating physiological differences
with assumptions about normal behavior
is known as _____.

10/42   * secondary sex character-
           istics
         Gender Identity
         Page #224

Deepening voice, facial hair, and
muscle development in adolescent men
are known as _____.

10/43   * What role do I want sex
           to play in my life at this
           time?
         * What are my values re-
           garding sexual relation-
           ships?
         * Will a sexual relation-
           ship enhance my feelings
           about myself and my partner?
         Intimacy
         Page #228

What are the three basic questions you
should ask yourself before getting
involved in a sexual relationship?
1. _____
2. _____
3. _____

Chapter 10: Sexuality

10/44   * accept feelings as they
          are
        * Use "I" statements
        * share your feelings
        * express interest and con-
          cern if your partner
          loses interest
        * speak up if something
          hurts during sex
        * state what you'd like to
          do differently
        * practice saying the words
          if you feel embarrassed
        * set aside regular time for
          discussions about sex
        Sexual Behavior
        Page #231

Discussing sex can be difficult. What are five ways to make this task easier?

1. _____
2. _____
3. _____
4. _____
5. _____

10/45   * sex is physically uncom-
          fortable or painful
        * sexual activity is con-
          stantly declining
        * you have a fear or revul-
          sion of sex
        * your sexual pleasure is
          declining
        * your sexual desire is
          diminishing
        * your sexual problems are
          increasing in frequency or
          intensity
        Problems
        Page #233

List four reasons to seek help with sexual problems.

1. _____
2. _____
3. _____
4. _____

<u>AN INVITATION TO HEALTH</u>
TEST BANK

Section III - Your Sexuality: Responsibility
and Rewards

<u>Chapter 11: Sexual Health</u>

In this chapter -

*   Sexual Health
*   Women's Health
*   Men's Health
*   Contraception
*   Abortion
*   Safe Sex

Section III - Your Sexuality: Responsibility
and Rewards
Chapter 11: Sexual Health

True-False

11/1	True Sexual Health Page #246	Responsible sexual relationships re-quire informed choices regarding dis-ease prevention and contraception.
11/2	False Women's Health Page #246	Problems associated with women's sexual health have been understood for cen-turies.
11/3	True Women's Health Page #246	Midway through the menstrual cycle, an egg is released during a process called ovulation.
11/4	False Women's Health Page #248	Dysmenorrhea is characterized by a cessation of the menstrual flow.
11/5	True Men's Health Pages #249-250	The most common benefit of circum-cision, the removal of the foreskin, is that it prevents oils and secretions from accumulating.
11/6	True Men's Health Page #250	Prostatitis, or infection of the pros-tate gland, is a common sexual problem in younger men.
11/7	False Men's Health Page #250	Enlargement of the prostate gland is caused by a diet high in zinc.
11/8	True Contraception Page #252	A sexually active couple that does not use contraception has an 80% chance of conceiving a child within 12 months.
11/9	True Contraception Page #256	Ideally, the decision about whether or not to use birth control, and/or which kind of contraception to use, should be made by both sexual partners.
11/10	False Contraception Page #252	Most sexually active teenage girls have an adequate understanding of the basics of contraception.
11/11	True Contraception Page #256	The basic issue regarding contraception for you and your partner is the impor-tance of not conceiving a child at this time in your lives.

11/12	True	Oral contraceptives interfere with the normal body chemistry of a woman as a means of preventing conception.
	Contraception	
	Page #256	

11/13	True	For women over 35, use of oral contraceptives increases the risk of cardiovascular problems such as stroke or heart attacks.
	Contraception	
	Page #256	

11/14	False	The major reason for the relatively low effectiveness rate for condoms is the low quality of materials used in production.
	Contraception	
	Page #259	

11/15	True	Use of barrier contraceptives has been shown to reduce the risk of infertility in women.
	Contraception	
	Page #258	

11/16	False	The Intrauterine Device (IUD) is a safe method of birth control when compared to the pill or barrier methods.
	Contraception	
	Page #260	

11/17	True	Sterilization is the most popular form of birth control among married couples in the United States.
	Contraception	
	Page #264	

11/18	False	The highest abortion rates in the U.S. are among women aged 15-17.
	Abortion	
	Page #269	

11/19	False	The health risks associated with sex have developed over the past 75 years.
	Safe Sex	
	Page #271	

11/20	False	AIDS is a homosexual disease.
	Safe Sex	
	Page #272	

Multiple Choice

11/21   a

Women's Health
Pages #247-248

Premenstrual syndrome

a. is a physiological problem probably caused by a hormonal deficiency or stress.
b. is a psychological condition indicating the beginning of menopause.
c. is characterized by mild symptoms of fatigue, irritability, headaches, and cravings for certain foods.
d. has no known treatment at this time.

11/22	d Women's Health Page #249	Menopause a. usually occurs between the ages of 45 and 55. b. is caused by increases in the level of estrogen in the woman's body. c. effects are limited to physical symptoms such as hot flashes or fatigue. d. is an experience that most women respond to negatively.
11/23	b Men's Health Page #250	Fever, pain during defecation, and pus in the urine are symptoms of a. male menopause. b. prostatitis. c. benign prostatic hypertrophy. d. prostate cancer.
11/24	c Men's Health Page #250	Changes in male sexual response that occur as a result of aging include longer arousal time, briefer orgasm, and a. shorter time before ejaculation. b. slower loss of erection following orgasm. c. smaller volume of ejaculate. d. decrease in length of refractory period (time needed between orgasms).
11/25	d Contraception Page #252	Which of the following statements regarding contraception is most accurate? a. Effective methods of contraception have existed for hundreds of years. b. The most important consideration in choosing a method of birth control is convenience. c. The condom is the oldest method of birth control. d. No single method of birth control is 100% safe, convenient, and effective.
11/26	c Contraception Pages #252-253	Which of the following is not an important criteria for choosing a method of birth control? a. availability of product b. effectiveness of method c. preference based on experience with previous partner d. assurance of fertility when use is discontinued

11/27   a
Contraception
Page #256

The three types of oral contraceptives available in the United States are the the combination pill, the mini pill, and the

a. multiphasic pill.
b. micro pill.
c. 6 month pill.
d. morning after pill.

11/28   b
Contraception
Page #256

Unlike women who take combination pills, those who take the mini pill

a. stop menstruating completely.
b. may ovulate occasionally.
c. are raising their estrogen levels.
d. achieve contraception through regulation of the ovulation and menstrual cycles.

11/29   c
Contraception
Pages #258-259

Which of the following is not a barrier contraceptive?

a. condom
b. cervical cap
c. intrauterine device
d. diaphragm

11/30   b
Contraception
Page #262

The major disadvantage of intrauterine devices is their

a. low level of effectiveness.
b. serious health risks.
c. poor reversibility (return to fertility).
d. high level of systemic complications compared to the pill.

11/31   d
Contraception
Page #262

Which of the following statements about vaginal spermicides is most accurate?

a. The side effects of vaginal spermicide use are serious.
b. All vaginal spermicides must be used with a diaphragm in order to be effective.
c. Foam is the least effective type of spermicidal product.
d. The spermicide nonoxynol-9 can kill the virus that causes AIDS.

11/32   a
         Contraception
         Page #266

The cervical mucus, calendar, and basal body temperature methods are all forms of birth control that rely (for their effectiveness) on

a. the timing of sexual intercourse.
b. the interruption of ovulation.
c. early withdrawal of the penis.
d. reduced sperm count levels in the male partner.

11/33   d
         Abortion
         Page #270

Methods of induced abortion include suction curettage, dilation and evacuation, and

a. vasectomy.
b. hysterectomy.
c. laparotomy.
d. hysterotomy.

11/34   d
         Abortion
         Page #270

The health risks of abortion

a. rise with the number of previous pregnancies.
b. remain constant throughout gestation (9 months of pregnancy).
c. should not prevent a couple from considering abortion as a practical and safe birth control alternative.
d. rise significantly after the first three months of pregnancy.

11/35   b
         Safe Sex
         Page #272

Acquired Immune Deficiency Syndrome (AIDS)

a. is a contagious disease spread by casual contact.
b. is not a disease itself, but a condition that weakens the body and makes it vulnerable to disease.
c. is primarily a disease of gay, white men.
d. is debilitating, but rarely fatal.

11/36   a
         Safe Sex
         Page #272

The AIDS virus is spread primarily

a. through the exchange of blood or other bodily fluids.
b. by sexual partners using barrier contraceptives.
c. through deep kissing and oral sex.
d. by sharing food, clothing, or dishes with an infected person.

Completion

11/37
* get plenty of exercise
* eat often and nutritiously
* get sufficient vitamins
* use less salt
* use less caffeine
* don't drink alcohol or smoke
* talk about your experience with a support group
Women's Health
Page #248

There are a number of things a woman can do to relieve premenstrual problems. List four of them.
1. _____
2. _____
3. _____
4. _____

11/38
* don't use tampons
* if you do use tampons, use "regular" instead of "superabsorbent"
* use napkins during the night and for some period during each day of menstrual flow
Women's Health
Page #248

List three ways to prevent toxic shock syndrome.
1. _____
2. _____
3. _____

11/39
* side effects of oral contraceptive use
Contraception
Page #257

Breakthrough bleeding, nausea, bloating, breast tenderness, and darkening of the skin across the nose and cheeks are all associated with _____.

11/40
* severe abdominal pain
* chest pain, coughing
* pain in calf or thigh
* severe headaches, dizziness or fainting
* muscle weakness/numbness
* speech disturbance
* eye problems
* breast lump
* severe depression
* yellowing skin
Contraception
Page #257-258

Use of oral contraceptives carries a degree of health risk. Identify five warning signs or symptoms that may indicate problems with oral contraceptive use.
1. _____
2. _____
3. _____
4. _____
5. _____

11/41
* Intrauterine Device (IUD)
Contraception
Page #260

Your friend has just come from a visit to her doctor to obtain birth control. In order to receive the form of birth control she desired, she had to sign a consent form acknowledging the posibility of surgery, sterility, permanent hormonal imbalance, and even death as a result of using the product. What form of birth control did she obtain?

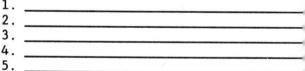

11/42   * during first cycle of
oral contraceptive use
* after forgetting to take
two or more pills, or
forgetting one pill during
the first week of the
menstrual cycle
* the first month after
switching to a different
brand of oral contraceptive
* when first learning to use
a diaphragm
Contraception
Page #264

There are certain times when no single
method of contraception may be sufficient to prevent conception. Identify two of them.
1. _____
2. _____

11/43   * effectiveness
* suitability to lifestyle
* side effects (if any)
* safety
* future fertility
* cost
* protection against
sexually transmitted dis-
ease
Contraception
Page #268

Choosing a method of contraception is
a decision best made with your partner.
Name four considerations important to
this critical decision.
1. _____
2. _____
3. _____
4. _____

11/44   * They are all birth control methods being tested
for future use

Contraception
Page #269

What do the following have in common:
Norplant, vaginal rings, testosterone
injections, Inhibin, and RU 486?

_____
_____

11/45   * IV drug use or sex with an
IV drug user
* sex with partners of unknown sexual history
* sex with people who re-
ceived blood transfusions
between 1978 and 1985.
* sex with anyone in certain
metropolitian areas
Safe Sex
Pages #272-273

Name four factors that increase your
chances of acquiring AIDS.
1. _____
2. _____
3. _____
4. _____

11/46   * anal receptive sex
         * sharing contaminated
           needles
         Safe Sex
         Pages #272-275

Homosexuals and IV drug users have been
identified very strongly with the AIDS
epidemic. Being gay or addicted will
not give you AIDS. Certain behaviors
associated with these two groups are
the major routes of transmission for
the AIDS virus. What are the two
behaviors most responsible for AIDS
transmission among members of these
two groups?

1. _____
2. _____

11/47   * Know all potential lovers
           as well as possible.
         * Limit the number of sex-
           ual partners.
         * Avoid sex practices that
           involve contact with
           semen or body fluids.
         * Males should wear a con-
           dom from beginning to
           end.
         * The woman should also use
           a diaphragm with
           nonoxynol-9 spermicide.
         Safe Sex
         Page #275

A relationship with a new friend is developing quickly, and might soon become
sexually intimate. What are three
things you can do to protect yourself
against sexually transmitted diseases?

1. _____
2. _____
3. _____

11/48   * the use of a condom
           treated with a spermi-
           cide containing
           nonoxynol-9
         Safe Sex
         Page #275

Barring abstinence what is the most
effective method of prevention against
the AIDS virus?

_____

<u>Matching</u>

11/49   Directions: Match each of the conception terms on the left with its
         correct definition on the right. Each definition may be used only
         once.

	<u>Term</u>	<u>Definition</u>
1.	__ spermatogenesis	a. merging of a ripe egg and sperm
2.	__ fertilization	b. the lining of the uterus
3.	__ ovulation	c. release of the egg by the ovary ·
4.	__ zygote	d. minute clump of cells formed from
5.	__ endometrium	the egg
6.	__ implantation	e. male sex cell
		f. creation of the sperm
		g. attachment of the cell clump to
		the lining of the uterus

         1-f, 2-a, 3-c,
         4-d, 5-b, 6-g
         Conception
         Pages #250-251

11/50   Directions: Match each of the sterilization techniques on the left
         with its correct description on the right. Each description may be
         used only once.

	<u>Technique</u>	<u>Description</u>
1.	__ tubal ligation	a. cutting of the vas deferens
2.	__ tubal occlusion	b. removal of the uterus
3.	__ laparotomy	c. cutting of the fallopian tubes,
4.	__ laparoscopy	usually following childbirth
5.	__ colpotomy	d. removal of the prostate gland
6.	__ hysterectomy	e. closing of the fallopian tubes via
7.	__ vasectomy	the vagina
		f. closing of the fallopian tubes
		using surgical instruments inserted
		through small opening in the abdo-
		men
		g. general term given to the blocking
		of the fallopian tubes
		h. general term given to the cutting
		or tying of the fallopian tubes

         1-h, 2-g, 3-c, 4-f,
         5-e, 6-b, 7-a
         Contraception
         Pages #264-266

Chapter 11: Sexual Health

<u>Essay</u>

11/51   Overpopulation and its attendant problems are foremost among the issues threatening the survival of our planet. Ironically, birth rates are often highest in those countries whose people can least afford to feed, house, and care for large families. How do you explain the reluctance of many Third World countries to embrace birth control and family planning?

11/52   In the U.S. birth control technology has focused primarily on the woman and her role in conception. Why hasn't there been more done to develop a "pill" for men?

11/53   The AIDS epidemic has forced our health care system to examine many of its values and assumptions about delivery of services, funding, and priorities. If you were Surgeon General of the United States, what steps would you take to deal with the AIDS crisis?

11/54   Abortion could become completely legal and state supported, or it could become outlawed totally and regarded as murder. What do you think the impact of these two extreme solutions would be on our society? Discuss each separately, and give examples of changes you might expect if they were a reality.

11/55   Safe sex is a term that will probably be with us for quite a while. What would you tell a young friend that came to you for advice about safe sex? Assume that your friend is of a different religion than you, and that you know little about their sexual behavior. How does your advice to your young friend differ from what you heard about sex when you were their age?

AN INVITATION TO HEALTH
TEST BANK

Section III - Your Sexuality: Responsibility
and Rewards

Chapter 12: Pregnancy and Parenting

In this chapter -

*   Choosing Children
*   Heredity
*   Pregnancy
*   Birthing
*   Infertility
*   Parenting

Section III - Your Sexuality: Responsibility
and Rewards
Chapter 12: Pregnancy and Parenting

True-False

12/1	True Choosing Children Page #280	According to mental health professionals, couples who decide not to have children are just as likely to be content with their marriage as those who do have children.
12/2	True Heredity Page #281	Traits and physical characteristics are passed on through generations by genes.
12/3	False Heredity Page #282	Genetic disorders are responsible for about 10 percent of all miscarriages.
12/4	False Pregnancy Page #286	The term "trimester" refers to the first three months of pregnancy.
12/5	True Pregnancy Page #286	Pregnancy tests are based on the presence of human chorionic gonadotropin (HCG) in the urine because it appears in a woman's body only during pregnancy.
12/6	False Pregnancy Page #287	Physiological changes caused by pregnancy become noticeable to the mother about six weeks after conception.
12/7	True Pregnancy Page #286	By the end of the third month, the fetus is completely formed.
12/8	False Pregnancy Page #286	Expectant mothers are usually most uncomfortable during the second trimester.
12/9	True Pregnancy Page #288	During pregnancy, fathers frequently experience mixed feelings about their changing roles.
12/10	True Pregnancy Page #292	Good prenatal care is critical to the health and well-being of both the mother and the baby.

Chapter 12: Pregnancy and Parenting

12/11	False Pregnancy Page #293	Smoking during pregnancy is a health risk for the mother, but not the baby.
12/12	True Pregnancy Page #297	Problems caused by high blood pressure are the most common form of medical complication during pregnancy.
12/13	False Birthing Page #300	There are four stages of labor.
12/14	False Infertility Page #305	Most often, infertility is the problem of the individual man or woman in a relationship.
12/15	True Parenting Page #312	Less than 20% of the 56 million families in the United States are conventional nuclear families.

Multiple Choice

12/16   b
Choosing Children
Page #280

Which of the following statements about having children is most accurate?

a. Less than 25% of all married couples say they plan to have children.
b. Having children because of immature or unrealistic reasons often places unreasonable burdens on the child.
c. Conceiving accidentally has not been shown to affect how couples view their relationship.
d. Fertility declines dramatically in a woman after age 25.

12/17   a
Heredity
Page #282

Traits carried by recessive genes are of concern to prospective parents because

a. they aren't manifest in either parent, but could become apparent in a child.
b. such traits are always fatal.
c. such traits are obvious in the parents, but shouldn't be passed on to the child.
d. there is a 75% chance that such traits will become manifest in the couple's children.

12/18 d
   Heredity
   Page #284

Amniocentesis is

a. a genetic problem common to Eastern European Jews.
b. an infection that occurs in the amniotic fluid of a pregnant woman.
c. a genetic disease caused by inbreeding.
d. a method of diagnosing genetic defects in a fetus.

12/19 c
   Pregnancy
   Page #286

Which of the following is not a common physiological change of the first trimester of pregnancy?

a. nausea or vomiting in the morning
b. fatigue
c. secretion of colostrum from the breasts
d. increased urination

12/20 a
   Pregnancy
   Page #287

Waste disposal and provision of nutrients to the fetus are functions performed by the

a. placenta.
b. amnion.
c. embryo.
d. zygote.

12/21 b
   Pregnancy
   Page #287

Which of the following descriptions most accurately characterizes a fetus at the end of the third month of development?

a. length is 4 inches, weight 2 ounces, movement can be felt by mother
b. length 2 inches, weight is 1/2 ounce, sex is differentiated
c. length is 1.2 inches, circulatory system is complete, fingers and toes are distinct
d. weight is 1.4 pounds, skin appears wrinkled, eyebrows and fingernails developed

12/22 c
   Pregnancy
   Page #289

Physiological changes occuring during the second trimester include weight gain, increase in heart size and blood volume, indigestion, and

a. Braxton-Hicks contractions.
b. pinching of the sciatic nerve.
c. secretion of colostrum from the breasts.
d. dropping of baby's head into the pelvis.

12/23   c
         Pregnancy
         Page #290

By the end of the second trimester
(6 months) the fetus

a. has a good chance of survival if
   born.
b. is about 8 inches long and is
   covered by lanugo.
c. is about one foot long with an
   immature respiratory system.
d. has smooth skin and weighs about
   4 pounds.

12/24   b
         Pregnancy
         Page #291

The end of fetal development is characterized by

a. formation and maturation of the
   heart.
b. preparation of the lungs for
   breathing.
c. sex differentiation.
d. production of the vernix.

12/25   d
         Pregnancy
         Page #292

A woman should have her first prenatal
visit with her doctor

a. at the end of the first trimester.
b. six weeks after conception.
c. as soon as she begins to feel un-
   comfortable.
d. as soon as she knows she is pregnant.

12/26   a
         Pregnancy
         Page #292

Current medical opinion states that the
nutritional supplements needed by a
pregnant woman are

a. folic acid and iron.
b. calcium and vitamin A.
c. vitamins C and D.
d. completely provided for in the
   average diet.

12/27   b
         Pregnancy
         Pages #293-294

The best advice to pregnant women
regarding smoking, alcohol, caffeine,
and drug use, is

a. not to exceed levels of use prior
   to becoming pregnant.
b. to avoid them all if possible.
c. cut back on alcohol consumption to
   3 ounces of alcohol per day.
d. not to worry because your baby is
   protected by the placenta.

12/28   c
Pregnancy
Page #296

Risk factors for ectopic pregnancy, or pregnancy outside the uterus, include previous surgery involving the fallopian tubes, pelvic inflammatory disease, infertility, and

a. use of oral contraceptives.
b. family history of miscarriages.
c. current use of an IUD.
d. being 35 years of age or older.

12/29   d
Teen Pregnancy
Page #298

Which of the following statements about pregnancy in the United States is <u>least</u> accurate?

a. The rate of teen pregnancy is the highest of all developed countries.
b. Nearly half of all black women become pregnant before the age of 20.
c. Teen pregnancy poses real health risks for both mother and child.
d. Teen pregnancy does not affect future economic or education opportunities.

12/30   c
Birthing
Pages #299-300

Current alternative approaches to the choice of birth attendants and site of delivery are characterized by

a. increased involvement by physicians.
b. high technology and medical intervention.
c. more active roles for the parents and emphasis on natural physiological processes.
d. increased use of new drugs.

12/31   a
Birthing
Page #301

Which of the following statements about labor is most accurate?

a. The actual birth of the baby occurs during the second stage.
b. The actual birth of the baby occurs during the third stage.
c. The transition phase is marked by less pain and easier contractions.
d. Braxton-Hicks contractions occur during the first stage.

12/32   b
Birthing
Page #302

Cesarean births

a. are routinely performed by licensed
midwives.
b. have more than doubled during the
past 10 years.
c. usually involve general anesthesia
(i.e., the mother is asleep).
d. prevent the mother from ever having
a vaginal delivery.

12/33   a
Birthing
Page #305

Which of the following is not an advantage of breast-feeding?

a. assurance that the milk is pure
b. enhanced bonding between mother and
child
c. healthier babies
d. convenience

12/34   c
Infertility
Pages #305-307

Infertility problems

a. are decreasing among the most fer-
tile group of women (ages 20-24).
b. among women are frequently psychological.
c. among men are usually related to the
quantity or quality of sperm.
d. can be diagnosed medically in only
about 50% of affected couples.

12/35   d
Infertility
Page #307

Extracting one or more ova from the
woman in order to fertilize it, and
then replacing the developing embryo
back into the mother's uterus is known
as

a. endometriosis.
b. artificial insemination.
c. embryo transfer.
d. in vitro fertilization.

12/36   b
Parenting
Pages #308-310

Effective parenting depends on

a. having at least one parent at home
during the day.
b. the ability of the parent(s) to
meet the child's basic needs.
c. both parents living together as a
nuclear family.
d. each parent adopting traditional
role behaviors and attitudes.

12/37   c
Parenting
Page #312

A child's adjustment to divorce depends primarily on the level of dis-
cord in the family prior to the
divorce and

a. the child's sex.
b. whether or not the child has any
   siblings.
c. the child's age.
d. which parent is at fault.

12/38   d
Parenting
Page #313

The three components of the child abuse
pattern include the potential for
abuse, a child who is perceived to be
different, and

a. a mentally ill parent.
b. low socio-economic status.
c. a parent who doesn't know his/her
   own strength.
d. a crisis or precipitating event.

Completion

12/39   * cystic fibrosis
Heredity
Page #283

The most common genetic problem among
American whites is a disabling abnormality of the respiratory system known
as _____.

12/38   * sickle-cell anemia
Heredity
Page #283

A genetic disorder affecting blacks
that affects the blood's ability to
transport oxygen (and kills half its
victims before the age of 20) is
called _____.

12/39   * consume 300 calories more
           each day when pregnant
         * do not restrict salt
         * drink six to eight glass-
           es of liquids each day
         * never diet during preg-
           nancy
         * eat the right foods -
           several servings per day
           from the major food groups
         * plan on a weight gain from
           20 to 30 pounds
Pregnancy
Page #292

Identify four of the nutritional guidelines for mothers-to-be developed by
the American College of Obstetrics and
Gynecology.
1. _____
2. _____
3. _____
4. _____

12/40
* exercise 3 times a week
* don't exercise strenuously for more than 15 minutes
* avoid exercising in hot, humid weather
* avoid jerky/bouncy motions
* stretch/flex carefully
* after the fourth month, don't exercise while lying flat on your back
* drink plenty of fluids
* don't let your body temperature rise above 100 F. or your heart rate climb above 140 beats/minute
* don't begin a new sport, play in moderation
* don't water-ski or surf
Pregnancy
Page #293

You have a pregnant friend who is concerned about fitness. Identify five exercise guidelines she should follow.
1. _____
2. _____
3. _____
4. _____
5. _____

12/41
* vaginal bleeding
* abdominal pain
* persistent nausea or vomiting
* unusual thirst
* chills or fever
* swelling of the face or fingers
* severe or continuous headaches
* dimness or blurring of vision
* fluid leaking from the vagina
Pregnancy
Page #298

Identify six warning signs of problems in pregnancy.
1. _____
2. _____
3. _____
4. _____
5. _____
6. _____

12/42
* experience in dealing with complications
* extensive prenatal care
* a commitment to be present during the entire labor
* a philosophy that is compatible with the parent's attitudes and values
Birthing
Page #299

A couple you know is considering alternatives to traditional birthing, and are looking for a midwife. Name three criteria they should use in their selection.
1. _____
2. _____
3. _____

12/43

* give praise and attention for good behavior, not bad
* spank only when the child is in danger
* look for the cause of the undesired behavior
* learn how to listen more and talk less
* when possible, offer the child two acceptable choices
* involve children in problem solving

Parenting
Page #311

Name four ways to be a better parent.

1. _____
2. _____
3. _____
4. _____

12/44

* the way the parent was reared
* extreme isolation leading to distrust or manipulation
* an extremely passive spouse
* poor self-images
* unrealistic expectations for the child

Parenting
Page #313

Identify three of the five factors that contribute to the potential for child abuse in parents.

1. _____
2. _____
3. _____

Chapter 12: Pregnancy and Parenting

Matching

12/45   Directions: Match each of the genetic terms on the left with its correct definition on the right. Each definition may be used only once.

Term	Definition
1. __ gene	a. when two genes for the same trait express themselves differently
2. __ chromosomes	b. rodlike structures within a cell that carry the genes
3. __ deoxyribonucleic acid/DNA	c. instructions for development of the fetus
4. __ homozygous	d. the number of chromosomes found in a gamete
5. __ heterozygous	e. a trait that is not apparent
6. __ dominant	f. the sex-determining chromosome
7. __ recessive	g. the number of chromosomes found in all cells except the egg and sperm
8. __ haploid	h. when two genes for the same trait express themselves similarly
9. __ diploid	i. what genes are made of
	j. a trait that is apparent

1-c, 2-b, 3-i, 4-h, 5-a,
6-j, 7-e, 8-d, 9-g
Heredity
Pages #281-282

Essay

12/46   "Test-tube babies" were once regarded as fantasies of science fiction writers. As science has advanced on the frontiers of conception and fertilization, many people question the moral, ethical, and spiritual implications of research in this area. What constraints, if any, do you think ought to be placed on research into conception and fertilization? Why? Defend your choices.

12/47   Surrogate parenting has received a great deal of media attention. Much of the discussion about surrogacy revolves around the validity of surrogacy contracts, and whether or not they are legally binding. Do you think surrogacy is a legitimate alternative for infertile couples? What are the primary advantages and disadvantages for those involved?

12/48   Adoption is now big business in many areas of the country. Private adoption agencies command huge fees for their services and still have long waiting lists. What was once a function of social service agencies has now grown into an international market. If you were able to regulate adoption proceedings, what regulations and guidelines would you impose? Why?

12/49   Less than one fifth of our nation's families can be considered traditional/nuclear (both parents living at home with their own children/no relatives in home). What do you think has contributed to the changing structure of families in America? Are the new family structures functional? If so, how? If not, why not?

12/50   Conceiving and raising children is probably the most demanding job most adults ever experience. Doing it well is even more difficult. What do you think of the idea that parents who agree to be trained and educated in parenting skills should be subsidized by the government for their time and labor? Why isn't the education and nurturing of a productive citizen worth as much to our country as the production of tobacco or the extraction of oil (both subsidized activities)?

<u>AN INVITATION TO HEALTH</u>
TEST BANK

Section IV - Your Lifestyle: Avoiding Harmful Habits

<u>Chapter 13: Drug Abuse</u>

In this chapter -

*   Use and Effects
*   Legal Abuse
*   Illegal Abuse
*   Psychoactive Drugs
*   Treatment

Section IV - Your Lifestyle: Avoiding Harmful Habits
Chapter 13: Drug Abuse

True-False

13/1   True
        Use and Effects
        Page #321

Caffeine, nicotine, and alcohol are all potentially addictive drugs.

13/2   False
        Use and Effects
        Page #321

Excessive use of drugs, in a way not acceptable to medical practice, is called drug misuse.

13/3   True
        Use and Effects
        Page #323

The term dependence refers to both the physical and psychological attachment that a person may develop to a drug.

13/4   True
        Legal Abuse
        Page #324

The average American consumes an amount of caffeine each day equivalent to 10-12 cans of soft drink.

13/5   False
        Legal Abuse
        Page #324

Painkillers such as aspirin and acetaminophen are examples of over-the-counter drugs that are rarely abused.

13/6   False
        Legal Abuse
        Page #325

The majority of drugs prescribed by physicians are used properly.

13/7   True
        Illegal Abuse
        Page #326

4 out of every 5 people over the age of 25 have tried an illegal drug.

13/8   False
        Illegal Abuse
        Page #327

The primary reason that people begin to take illegal drugs is that the drugs are readily available.

13/9   True
        Illegal Abuse
        Page #330

Polyabuse, or the use of multiple illegal drugs, increases the chances of harmful side effects.

13/10   True
        Psychoactive Drugs
        Page #330

Drugs that affect the central nervous system are known as psychoactive drugs.

13/11   False
        Psychoactive Drugs
        Page #331

Cocaine is not addictive.

13/12	True Psychoactive Drugs Page #331	Cocaine use produces feelings of euphoria, energy, mental awareness, and a false sense of increased muscular strength.
13/13	True Psychoactive Drugs Page #333	Prolonged use of cocaine is now considered at least as deadly as heroin.
13/14	True Psychoactive Drugs Page #333	Amphetamine dependence occurs when a user must continue to take increasingly larger amounts in order to prevent the depression that follows when the drug wears off.
13/15	True Psychoactive Drugs Page #334	The most widely used sedative is alcohol.
13/16	False Psychoactive Drugs Page #334	Barbiturates are rarely involved in drug-related deaths.
13/17	False Psychoactive Drugs Page #336	Because marijuana is a plant and not a processed chemical, users don't have to worry about dangerous substances or contamination.
13/18	True Psychoactive Drugs Page #337	LSD is about 1000 times more potent than cocaine or hashish.
13/19	False Psychoactive Drugs Pages #338-340	Opium, morphine, codeine, and heroin are all products of the hemp plant.
13/20	True Treatment Page #343	Effective and enduring drug rehabilitation depends on the abuser's ability to rebuild a network of social contacts who will help him/her with recovery.

Multiple Choice

13/21   a
         Use and Effects
         Page #321

The physiological effects of drugs on the body depend on the method of drug introduction into the body, the drug's action, and

a. the presence of other drugs in the body.
b. whether or not the person is addicted.
c. the user's motives for taking the drug.
d. the user's knowledge of drug effects.

13/22   c
Legal Abuse
Page #325

Which of the following statements about prescription drugs is <u>least</u> accurate?

a. About 50% of all drugs prescribed each year are improperly used.
b. 10 to 20 percent of hospital admissions are related to prescription drug misuse.
c. Steroids are a form of amphetamines.
d. Prolonged use of amphetamines can cause a form of paranoia called amphetamine psychosis.

13/23   b
Illegal Abuse
Page #327

Which of the following statements about drug dependency is most accurate?

a. Stage 2 is marked by a preoccupation with getting high and unpredictable behavior.
b. Drug dependency must be viewed against a background of a pleasure-prizing society and ambivalent attitudes toward drugs.
c. A user is hooked when he/she experiences the feeling of euphoria caused by drugs.
d. Early drug use is marked by efforts to avoid psychological or physical pain.

13/24   d
Psychoactive Drugs
Pages #331-332

Cocaine's effect on the brain and body include impaired judgement, seizures, severe loss of appetite, and

a. enhanced sexual desire.
b. increased muscular strength.
c. improved mental alertness lasting several hours per dose.
d. heart attacks.

13/25   b
Psychoactive Drugs
Page #332

Cocaine

a. produces ill effects only when inhaled.
b. can seriously harm the baby of a woman who uses the drug while she's pregnant.
c. habits, when compared to other drugs, are relatively easy to break.
d. dependence affects only about 1% of all cocaine users.

13/26   c
Psychoactive Drugs
Page #333

Amphetamine abuse occurs primarily by users seeking to

a. lessen fatigue.
b. improve concentration.
c. get high, or experience euphoria.
d. improve physical performance.

13/27   d
Psychoactive Drugs
Page #334

Which of the following statements about sedatives is <u>not</u> accurate?

a. Sedatives all affect behavior in the same way.
b. When mixed together, sedatives have a synergistic effect.
c. As you develop a tolerance for one sedative, you also develop tolerance for other sedatives.
d. Barbiturates cannot cross the pla- placenta and harm the fetus.

13/28   a
Psychoactive Drugs
Page #335

Antianxiety medications

a. are the most widely prescribed drugs the United States.
b. are absorbed quickly into the bloodstream.
c. do not have a synergistic effect when combined with alcohol.
d. have a mild synergistic effect when combined with alcohol that is <u>not</u> life threatening.

13/29   a
Psychoactive Drugs
Page #336

Marijuana use

a. produces effects on the central nervous system similar to alcohol when consumed at low to moderate doses.
b. produces physical dependency.
c. is no longer federally regulated.
d. cannot really be considered a "gateway" drug.

13/30   c
Psychoactive Drugs
Page #336

Regular use of marijuana results in central nervous system impairment, increases in heart rate, damage to the lungs, and

a. enhanced coordination.
b. higher levels of motivation.
c. possible reproductive system damage.
d. heightened immune response.

13/31   d
Psychoactive Drugs
Page #337

Mescaline and psilocybin belong to a class of drugs known as psychedelics that, when taken, produce

a. extreme physical reactions.
b. lethargy and sleepiness.
c. tolerance for pain and stress.
d. hallucinations and altered perceptions of reality.

13/32   b
Psychoactive Drugs
Page #338

The major drawback to the use of psychedelics and drugs like PCP is

a. their potential for addiction.
b. their behavioral toxicity and unpredictable effects.
c. their synergistic effect when mixed with sedatives.
d. their relatively short period of effect, leading to increasingly frequent use.

13/33   c
Psychoactive Drugs
Page #338

Narcotics

a. is a term used to refer to all illicit drugs.
b. have a low potential for abuse and dependency.
c. dependency is very likely with frequent or long-term use.
d. withdrawal lasts about 24 hours.

13/34   a
Psychoactive Drugs
Page #340

Which of the following statements about heroin is most accurate?

a. Over two million people in the United States are addicted to heroin.
b. Heroin is now a suburban drug, most popular among affluent whites.
c. The effects of heroin last about eight to ten hours.
d. Tolerance to heroin develops slowly.

13/35   b
Psychoactive Drugs
Page #340

Synthetic narcotics

a. are not addictive.
b. have been used to help heroin addicts stop taking heroin.
c. are rarely overdosed, and cause fewer deaths each year than heroin.
d. cannot be abused.

13/36   d
            Psychoactive Drugs
            Page #341

Inhalants such as glue, cleaning fluid, and butane, can cause serious medical problems such as liver and kidney failure, muscle and bone destruction, blood abnormalities, and

a. enhanced mental functions.
b. hallucinations.
c. improved coordination.
d. potentially fatal, irregular heart-beats.

13/37   b
            Consequences
            Page #342

Which of the following statements about drugs on the job is <u>least</u> accurate?

a. Cocaine is the primary drug of abuse on the job.
b. Job-related drug abuse is almost completely confined to the sports and entertainment business.
c. 5% to 13% of the U.S. work force abuses drugs other than alcohol.
d. Drug abuse costs more than $60 billion per year in treatment and lost productivity.

13/38   c
            Treatment
            Page #343

Successful drug treatment programs

a. have a success rate of about 25-30%
b. should be started as soon as a person has become physically or psychologically dependent.
c. involve a lifelong commitment.
d. have experienced stable demand over the past 5 years.

Completion

13/39   * name of the drug and its effects
            * how it should be taken, and when
            * what food, drinks, medicines, or activities should be avoided
            * what the side effects are, and how are they treated
            * what written information is available about the drug
            * is there an alternative treatment that might be equally effective
            Legal Abuse
            Page #325

What should you know about a drug that is prescribed by your doctor? Identify four kinds of information you should have.

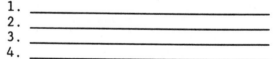

1. _____
2. _____
3. _____
4. _____

13/40
* learn how to cope with stress
* strengthen your self-esteem through involvement with activities you are good at
* develop a range of interests for relaxing
* practice assertiveness, speak up about what you believe in
Illegal Abuse
Pages #326-327

List three strategies for protecting yourself from the temptation to take drugs.
1. _____
2. _____
3. _____

13/41
* show/tell them you aren't interested
* have something else to do
* be prepared for pressure
* keep your "no" simple
* ignore the offer
* change the subject
* hang out with people who don't use drugs
Illegal Abuse
Page #327

Identify four ways to say "no" to someone who offers you drugs.
1. _____
2. _____
3. _____
4. _____

13/42
* abrupt change in attitude, moodiness
* sudden decline in school attendance or performance
* resistance to discipline or criticism
* demands for secrecy or privacy that seem unreasonable
* changes in sleeping, eating habits; weight loss
* evidence of drug use (odor, paraphernalia)
* borrowing of money, stealing
* lack of interest in family
* temper flare-ups, poor appearance
* friendships with known drug users
Illegal Abuse
Page #328

Your friend Peter approaches you with a concern about his sister. She's hanging out with a new group of friends and Peter is worried about drugs. Name 6 warning signals Peter should be looking for.
1. _____
2. _____
3. _____
4. _____
5. _____
6. _____

13/43   Alcohol: affects perception, coordination, increases effects of sedatives
Marijuana: affects ability to brake, stay in lane, slows thinking and re-flexes, lasts 4-6 hours
Tranquilizers: slow reac-tion time and impair judgement
Sedatives: make driver sleepy, can have "morning after" effect
Stimulants: impair coor-dination
Hallucinogens: distorted judgement and reality, cause severe panic, confusion, mental problems
Illegal Abuse
Page #342

For each of the drugs listed below, identify the effect that use has on driving ability.

Alcohol: _____

Marijuana: _____

Tranquilizers: _____

Sedatives: _____

Stimulants: _____

Hallucinogens: _____

13/44   a) the supervised withdrawal from drug dependence
b) highly structured, drug-free environments that rely on group therapy and peer pressure for re-covery
c) programs that emphasize counseling and faith in a higher power to sup-port recovery
Treatment
Page #343

Define each of the following terms: a) detoxification, b) therapeutic communities, and c) outpatient drug-free program.
a) _____

b) _____

c) _____

Matching

13/45   Directions: Match each of the terms on the left with its correct
         definition on the right.   Each definition may be used only once.

	Term		Definition
1.	__ additive		a. the body's ability to withstand the effects of a drug
2.	__ synergistic		b. the interaction of two drugs produces an effect greater than the sum of the two drugs taken at different times
3.	__ potentiating		
4.	__ antogonistic		c. heightened effect of a drug because it is taken in faster than the body can metabolize or excrete it
5.	__ toxicity		
6.	__ tolerance		d. the effect caused by drugs that neutralize or block each other with opposite effects
			e. interaction between drugs equal to the sum of the effects of the drugs used
			f. one drug increasing the effect of the other
			g. the level at which a drug becomes poisonous to the body

1-e, 2-b, 3-f,
4-d, 5-g, 6-a
Use and Effects
Page #323

Essay

13/46   Everyone seems to be concerned about the "drug problem." Yet many
         people oppose the location of drug treatment facilities such as
         halfway houses in their community. What kinds of concerns do you
         think people like this have? Are they legitimate? How would you deal
         with resistance to community-based drug treatment?

13/47   What role do you think over-the-counter (OTC) drug manufacturers and
         their lobbyists play in the drug problem, if any? If the drug problem
         is so critical, why are these companies allowed to continue to promote
         the idea that drug use is a safe and reasonable approach to stress
         management, worries, anxiety, etc.? If you were in a position to
         regulate the commerce and promotion of OTC products, what changes
         would you make? Defend your choices.

13/48   Legalization of currently illegal drugs has been proposed as a means
         of bringing our drug problem under control. What are the arguments
         for and against such an approach?

13/49   Much of the debate about our nation's drug habit deals with the
         questions of where we should spend our limited resources: enforcement
         of drug laws or treatment and education. If it were up to you, how
         would you divide up resources made available to combat drug abuse?
         What data, if any, do you have to support your decisions?

13/50   Worksite testing for drug use is now commonplace. What worksites or
         jobs do you think <u>need</u> drug testing? Why? What criteria should be
         used to decide when and where worksite drug testing will be
         implemented?

AN INVITATION TO HEALTH
TEST BANK

Section IV - Your Lifestyle: Avoiding Harmful Habits

Chapter 14: Alcohol

In this chapter -

* Consumption
* Moderation
* Effects
* Alcoholism

Section IV - Your Lifestyle: Avoiding Harmful Habits
Chapter 14: Alcohol

True-False

14/1	True Consumption Page #348	Alcohol is the most widely abused drug in the United States.
14/2	True Consumption Page #348	Among all illnesses, alcohol-related diseases are the second leading cause of death and disability.
14/3	False Consumption Page #348	Most adults in the U.S. drink moderately (more than three alcoholic drinks per week).
14/4	True Consumption Page #349	Alcohol is the most frequently used drug on college campuses.
14/5	False Consumption Page #349	Alcoholism is not a significant drug problem among young people in the U.S.
14/6	False Consumption Page #350	The amount (volume) of alcoholic beverage consumed by an individual is the most accurate measure of actual alcohol consumption.
14/7	True Moderation Page #351	Moderate drinkers tend to be healthier than both alcoholics and those who abstain altogether.
14/8	True Moderation Page #351	Your liver is capable of metabolizing about 0.5 ounce of alcohol every hour.
14/9	False Effects Page #353	The rate at which alcohol is metabolized by the body is dependent on the amount of alcohol consumed.
14/10	True Effects Page #356	The organ most vulnerable to chronic alcohol abuse is the liver.
14/11	False Effects Page #357	Alcohol stimulates the central nervous system.

14/12 True
   Effects
   Page #358

Many frequently prescribed drugs have at least one ingredient that interacts adversely with alcohol.

14/13 True
   Effects
   Page #359

Consumption of alcohol, particularly more than three drinks per week, significantly increases a woman's chances of contracting breast cancer.

14/14 False
   Alcoholism
   Page #360

Alcoholism affects 25 out of every 100 people who use alcohol.

14/15 True
   Alcoholism
   Page #361

Alcoholism is characterized primarily by loss of control over the use and impact of alcohol.

14/16 False
   Alcoholism
   Page #361

The norms and values of a society have little impact on the rate of alcoholism.

14/17 True
   Alcoholism
   Page #363

Alcohol-related diseases are responsible for almost 50% of all hospital admissions.

14/18 False
   Alcoholism
   Pages #363-365

Compared to other diseases, alcoholism's cost to society is relatively low.

14/19 True
   Alcoholism
   Page #366

The greatest barrier to recovery from alcoholism is denial of the illness.

14/20 False
   Alcoholsim
   Page #368

Most recovered alcoholics go on to be stable, moderate drinkers.

Mulitple Choice

14/21 d
   Consumption
   Page #348

2 X

Analysis of recent patterns of alcohol consumption reveals that

a. sales of beer have increased.
b. wine sales have fallen.
c. almost one half of all adults abstain entirely from drinking alcohol.
d. only 1 in 10 adults drink one ounce or more of alcohol per day.

14/22 b
Consumption
Page #348

Which of the following statements about alcohol consumption is most accurate?

a. Women of all ages are more likely to drink than men.
b. Heavy and moderate drinkers are more likely to be found in upper socio-economic levels.
c. The average age at which children take their first drink is 15 years.
d. Most college students do not drink.

14/23 c
Consumption
Page #349

The most common reason people drink is

a. to emulate people they admire.
b. because they are manipulated by advertising.
c. to relax.
d. because they are embarrassed to say "no."

14/24 a
Consumption
Page #350

Each of the following drinks contains about 0.5 ounce of alcohol except one. Which one is it?

a. a 16 ounce can of malt liquor that is 12 proof
b. a scotch and soda with one ounce of 100 proof scotch whiskey
c. a 4 ounce glass of 24 proof table wine
d. a 12 ounce can of beer with 4.8% alcohol.

14/25 a
Consumption
Page #351

Which of the following is not one of three main patterns of chronic alcohol abuse?

a. exclusively drinking liquor or distilled spirits instead of wine or beer
b. regular heavy drinking on weekends
c. long periods of sobriety, followed by binges of heavy drinking
d. regular daily intake of large amounts of alcohol

14/26 b
Moderation
Page #352

Your friend Juan, who weighs 165 pounds, has consumed 6 glasses of table wine in the past two hours. He's had nothing to eat. Juan's blood alcohol concentration is probably

a. 0.01 percent
b. 0.10 percent
c. 0.50 percent
d. 1.00 percent

161

Chapter 14: Alcohol

14/27   c
         Moderation
         Page #352

Blood alcohol concentration (BAC) is a
measure of the amount of alcohol in the
bloodstream. It is also used to determine legal intoxication, which in most
states is

a. 0.01 percent BAC.
b. 0.05 percent BAC.
c. 0.10 percent BAC.
d. 0.25 percent BAC.

14/28   d
         Effects
         Page #355

6X

Which of the following statements about
the effects of alcohol consumption is
least accurate?

a. Blood alcohol content usually peaks
   about one hour after ingestion.
b. Alcohol is metabolized at a relatively constant rate.
c. Alcohol increases the rate at which
   fluids are eliminated from the body.
d. Most of the alcohol you drink leaves
   your body without being metabolized.

14/29   c
         Effects
         Page #357

X7

Which of the following statements most
accurately describes the relationship
between alcohol consumption and cardiovascular health?

a. Chronic alcohol use boosts the production of white blood cells.
b. Moderate alcohol consumption lowers
   blood pressure.
c. Moderate drinkers are less likely to
   be hospitalized with heart problems
   than those who have less than one
   drink per month.
d. Alcohol use has not been associated
   with weakened heart muscle.

14/30   b
         Effects
         Pages #357-358

X8

Alcohol affects perception and judgement in all but one of the following
ways. Which statement is not accurate?

a. Alcohol interferes with the body's
   ability to regulate its temperature.
b. Consumption of alcohol enhances
   reaction time and spatial judgement.
c. Drinking interferes with your
   ability to distinguish sounds.
d. Alcohol interferes with a man's
   ability to maintain an erection.

14/31   a
         Effects
         Page #359

Alcohol use by women increases their risk of breast cancer, damage to the fetus if they are pregnant, and

a. osteoporosis, or bone deterioration caused by calcium loss.
b. loss of cognitive skills and intellectual performance.
c. reduced levels of fertility.
d. earlier onset of menopause.

14/32   c
         Alcoholism
         Page #361

The definition of alcoholism as a disease is related most closely to

a. the total amount of alcohol consumed during an average day.
b. the blood alcohol content (BAC) after having a certain number of drinks.
c. the level of interference in one's life caused by the effects of alcohol consumption.
d. the presence of liver damage and other physical signs.

14/33   c
         Alcoholism
         Page #361

Which of the following factors has not been shown to be associated with alcoholism?

a. heredity
b. stress
c. moral character
d. cultural norms

14/34   d
         Alcoholism
         Page #363

Jaundice (yellow-appearing skin) and edema (swelling) of the hands and feet are signs of

a. alcohol intoxication.
b. alcohol poisoning.
c. malnutrition resulting from alcoholism.
d. liver damage.

14/35   d
         Alcoholism
         Page #363

Each year, alcoholism costs our society about

a. $17 million.
b. $117 million.
c. $17 billion.
d. $117 billion.

14/36   a
         Alcoholism
         Page #365

It is common for a child to respond to a parent's drinking by

a. becoming overly responsible and taking over many household tasks.
b. confronting the parent with the harmful impact of his/her drinking.
c. turning to alcohol abuse as a means of coping.
d. ignoring the problem completely.

14/37   c
         Treatment
         Page #366

Detoxification

a. is a form of treatment to help alcoholics overcome their psychological addiction to alcohol.
b. usually results in delusion and hallucinations (delirium tremens).
c. usually precedes treatment for psychological addiction.
d. produces withdrawal symptoms that last about 24 hours.

14/38   b
         Treatment
         Page #367

Alcoholics Anonymous, possibly the most effective means of treating alcoholism and maintaining sobriety, is based on the belief that

a. alcoholism is not really a disease.
b. alcoholics are powerless to control their drinking.
c. most alcoholics can learn to be moderate, social drinkers.
d. recovery from alcoholism takes about 2 years.

14/39   d
         Treatment
         Page #368

According to psychiatrist George Vaillant, recovery from alcoholism requires finding a substitute for alcohol and

a. avoiding people who drink.
b. avoiding stressful situations.
c. developing a strong sense of will-power.
d. developing an internal sense of self-esteem and hope.

<u>Completion</u>

14/40   * set a limit (2 drinks per day) and stick to it
* learn to say no simply
* drink slowly, enjoy all aspects of the experience
* don't drink your quota at a single sitting - spread them out during the week
* always eat before a party
* always use designated drivers (someone who will not drink at all) when you go out
* don't drink alone
Consumption
Page #351

Identify four strategies for insuring that you drink moderately.
1. _____
2. _____
3. _____
4. _____

14/41   * always measure the alcohol when you mix drinks
* drink slowly, never more than one per hour
* eat prior to, and during, drinking. Eat foods high in protein.
* avoid fizzy mixers like club soda.
Moderation
Page #354

State three things you can do to avoid getting drunk when you drink.
1. _____
2. _____
3. _____

14/42   * small head
* abnormal facial features
* poor muscle tone
* failure to thrive
* slow motor development
* sleep disorders
* short stature
* mental retardation
* hyperactivity
Effects
Page #359

Mothers who drink put their babies at risk for fetal alcohol syndrome. What are 5 symptoms of this condition?
1. _____
2. _____
3. _____
4. _____
5. _____

14/43
* symptoms after drinking
  including headaches, gas,
  nausea, or muscle cramps
* needing a drink to start
  the day
* denial of a problem
* doing things while drinking one later regrets
* dramatic mood swings
* sleep problems
* depression and paranoia
* forgetting about drinking
  episodes
* going on the wagon to control drinking
* having more than 5 drinks
  per day
Alcoholism
Page #361

You're concerned about a friend's involvement with alcohol. Identify six
warning signs of alcohol abuse.
1. _____
2. _____
3. _____
4. _____
5. _____
6. _____

14/44
* remain calm, unemotional
  and honest about the
  drinker's behavior
* discuss the situation with
  someone you trust
* include the drinker in
  family/friend's activities
* be patient, live one day
  at a time
* refuse to ride with the
  drinker when she/he is
  intoxicated
* never make excuses for the
  drinker
* don't assume responsibili-
  ties for the drinker
Alcoholism
Page #365

What are four things you can do if
someone you are close to drinks too
much?
1. _____
2. _____
3. _____
4. _____

Essay

14/46   In spite of all that is known about the harmful effects of alcohol
         abuse, we seem determined to protect our "right" to drink.
         Prohibition and regulation have not been successful in stemming the
         tide of alcohol abuse in this country. What steps do you think
         federal, state, and local governments could take in order to reduce
         our level of alcohol abuse?

14/47   Debate continues as to whether or not alcoholism is truly a disease,
         and whether or not alcoholics are responsible for their drinking. One
         recent argument is that the disease model of alcoholism is merely a
         reflection of our society's expectation that medicine has a cure for
         everything. What do you think would happen to our society if
         alcoholics were held responsible for their drinking behavior? What
         would be the social, legal, and cultural consequences of treating
         alcoholism not as a disease, but as willful misbehavior?

14/48   Many people who drink may not be aware of the possible health
         consequences of their behavior. Do you think liquor, beer, and wine
         should have warning labels? If so, what should they say? Write a
         warning label you would like to see on a bottle of 100 proof bourbon;
         a six pack of beer; a bottle of red wine.

14/49   Cultures that incorporate alcohol consumption into special events,
         rituals, formal ceremonies and other structured situations seem to
         have lower levels of abuse than those that view drinking as an
         independent activity. Do you believe that drinking alcohol in
         connection with a particular custom is more legitimate or less risky
         than drinking merely to relax? Why?

14/50   Take a position on the following statement and defend your point of
         view.

         "The expense of alcoholism ($100+ billion per year) should be
         recovered through a special tax on alcoholic beverages, with the money
         used for treatment and education programs."

Section IV - Your Lifestyle: Avoiding Harmful Habits

<u>Chapter 15: Tobacco</u>

In this chapter -

*   Smoking Today
*   Smoke Contents
*   Effects
*   Expense
*   Alternatives
*   Passive Smoking
*   Quitting

Section IV - Your Lifestyle: Avoiding Harmful Habits
Chapter 15: Tobacco

True-False

15/1   True
Smoking Today
Page #373

Tobacco use is responsible for most of the preventable deaths that occur in the U.S. each year.

15/2   False
Smoking Today
Page #373

Even though the population has grown, the actual number of smokers has decreased during the last two decades.

15/3   True
Smoking Today
Page #373

Most people who smoke believe that smoking in the workplace should be restricted to designated areas.

15/4   True
Smoking Today
Page #373

Black men between the ages of 25 and 34 comprise the highest percentage of smokers.

15/5   False
Smoking Today
Page #374

Most Americans are unaware that there are health risks associated with smoking.

15/6   True
Smoking Today
Page #375

According to recent research, cigarette smoking reduces anxiety and improves memory.

15/7   True
Smoking Today
Page #375

90% of all smokers are addicted to tobacco.

15/8   True
Smoking Today
Page #373

Tobacco is the most widespread addiction in the world.

15/9   False
Smoke Contents
Page #376

The addictive element in tobacco smoke is tar.

15/10   True
Effects
Page #378

Heart attacks are the leading cause of excessive deaths among smokers.

15/11   True
Effects
Page #379

Smoking is responsible for about 80% of all cases of lung cancer.

Chapter 15: Tobacco

15/12	False Expense Page #382	The U.S. government spends more each year convincing people <u>not</u> to smoke than tobacco companies spend on advertisements promoting their products.
15/13	False Alternatives Page #383	Alternative forms of tobacco use such as snuff do not pose serious health risks.
15/14	False Alternatives Page #383	Smokeless tobacco does not lead to nicotine addiction.
15/15	True Passive Smoking Page #386	Sidestream smoke (smoke not inhaled by the smoker) is more hazardous to a nonsmoker's health than mainstream smoke (smoke inhaled by the smoker).
15/16	True Passive Smoking Page #387	Most states now have laws prohibiting smoking in public places.
15/17	True Quitting Page #388	Young smokers who inhale deeply lose a minute of life for every minute they spend smoking.
15/18	False Quitting Page #388	After one year, only 10% of those who tried to quit are still not smoking.
15/19	False Quitting Page #388	Nicotine addiction is relatively easy to overcome compared to other drugs.
15/20	True Quitting Page #388	Most quitting techniques work best with a support group.

Multiple Choice

15/21	a Smoking Today Page #373	Which of the following statements about people who smoke is most accurate?

a. The higher their socioeconomic status, the less likely they are to smoke.
b. The age is rising at which smokers light up their first cigarette.
c. The later you start smoking, the more likely you are to be a heavy smoker.
d. Boys in their senior year of high school are more likely to smoke than their female peers.

15/22   c
Smoking Today
Page #374

Most people start to smoke cigarettes because

a. of the pleasant experience they have with the first few cigarettes.
b. they are genetically inclined to smoke.
c. they are curious, and there are strong social pressures to try it.
d. they want to lose weight.

15/23   b
Smoking Today
Page #374

With regard to the health risks associated with smoking, research done by the Federal Trade Commission shows that

a. the majority of Americans know that cigarette smoking can cause heart disease.
b. half of all women don't know that smoking increases the risk of still-birth or miscarriage.
c. 50% of those polled didn't know that smoking causes 80% of all lung cancer.
d. most Americans are not aware that there are health risks associated with smoking.

15/24   d
Smoking Today
Page #375

Most people continue to smoke because

a. they don't really want to stop.
b. they want to stop, but don't have the willpower to do it.
c. they have a low level of regard for themselves.
d. they are dependent on nicotine for feelings of pleasure.

15/25   c
Smoking Today
Page #376

The ways in which nicotine causes addiction include providing a strong experience of pleasure, producing severe discomfort during withrawal, and

a. interfering with the smoker's ability to understand the health risks.
b. raising the anxiety level of the smoker.
c. stimulating long-term cravings for a cigarette, even when the smoker has quit.
d. making food taste better.

15/26   b
Smoke Contents
Page #376

When a smoker inhales cigarette smoke, the nicotine

a. has a relatively consistent and stable effect.
b. is almost completely absorbed into the body.
c. acts to decrease blood pressure.
d. absorbed into the body is only about 25% of the amount present in the smoke.

15/27   d
Effects
Page #378

Which of the following statements about the health effects of smoking is not accurate?

a. A smoker is 10 times more likely to develop lung cancer than a non-smoker.
b. Smokers are 20 times more likely to have a heart attack than nonsmokers.
c. Lung cancer risks rise dramatically when smokers are exposed to asbestos.
d. The increased risk of heart attack caused by smoking never decreases, even if you quit smoking.

15/28   a
Effects
Page #379

Lung cancer

a. now kills more women than breast cancer.
b. has one of the best survival rates for any type of cancer.
c. is the third leading cause of cancer deaths in the U.S.
d. risk is related to how much people smoke, but not how long they smoke or when they started.

15/29   c
Effects
Page #379

The effect of cigarette smoke on the respiratory system is

a. rather slow, and takes about 5-10 years to become evident.
b. less dangerous than most other air-borne pollutants.
c. to progressively limit the flow of air into and out of the lungs.
d. reduced when the smoker is also exposed to other air pollutants.

15/30   d
Effects
Page #380

The health risks to women from smoking cigarettes

a. have declined because women who smoke today smoke fewer cigarettes per day than women ten years ago.
b. include higher chances of a heart attack, but only for those smoking more than 4 cigarettes per day.
c. are limited to respiratory and cancer related illnesses.
d. include increased incidence of miscarriage and pregnancy complications.

15/31   b
Costs
Page #382

During his/her lifetime, the amount of money spent on cigarettes by an average smoker is about

a. $1,500.
b. $15,000.
c. $25,000.
d. $50,000.

15/32   a
Alernatives
Page #383

Which of the following statements about alternative forms of tobacco is most accurate?

a. Clove cigarettes have twice as much nicotine and tar as moderate-tar American brands.
b. The risk of mouth and throat cancer to pipe smokers is lower than for cigarette smokers.
c. Smokeless tobacco is a safe substitute for smoking cigarettes.
d. The risks posed by snuff and chewing tobacco are not affected by the number of years they are used.

15/33   c
Passive Smoking
Page #386

The increased risk of lung cancer to a nonsmoker living with a smoker (over a lifetime) is

a. negligible.
b. twofold.
c. threefold.
d. fourfold.

15/34   d
        Passive Smoking
        Page #387

        X 19

Which of the following organizations
is most likely to dispute research
findings that reveal health risks to
passive smokers?

a. The American Lung Association
b. Action on Smoking and Health
c. The American Heart Association
d. The Tobacco Institute

15/35   c
        Passive Smoking
        Page #387

        X 20

Opponents of restrictions on smoking
at the worksite

a. agree that smoking interferes with
   performance.
b. agree that smoking poses specific
   health risks to nonsmokers, but that
   the risks are not significant.
c. argue that research regarding health
   risks to nonsmokers is not conclusive.
d. have conclusive evidence to support
   their argument that passive smoking
   is not harmful to nonsmokers.

15/36   b
        Quitting
        Page #388

The major advantage of stop-smoking
groups is that

a. they increase the success rate after
   one year from 25% to about 40%.
b. they can reduce the number of relapses quitters may experience.
c. they function as a substitute for
   the desire to quit that is absent
   in most smokers.
d. the success rates they advertise are
   backed up by the Federal Government.

Completion

15/37   * you are unable to stop
          smoking or significantly
          reduce the amount of to-
          bacco you use
        * when you stop using tobac-
          co, you develop withdrawal
          symptoms (headache, crav-
          ing for tobacco, anxiety)
        * you continue to use
          tobacco despite a serious
          physical problem that's
          worsened by tobacco
        * you resume tobacco use
          after quitting
        Smoking Today
        Page #376

What are three signs of tobacco addiction?
1. _____
2. _____
3. _____

15/38
* keep a record of your smokeless tobacco use
* gradually reduce the amount of time you keep tobacco in your cheek - brush afterwards
* use sugarless gum as a substitute
* find out what your friends (opposite sex) think of people who use smokeless tobacco
* when you're ready to quit, have your teeth cleaned
* drink a lot of fluids and exercise regularly to rid your body of nicotine

Alternatives
Page #386

What are four things you can do to stop using smokeless tobacco?
1. _____
2. _____
3. _____
4. _____

15/39
* let your friend know you support the decision
* offer to help with routine chores during the first few, tense days
* help your friend stay away from smokers and tobacco
* give up something yourself as a sign of support
* be prepared for problems with the relationship, try to forgive in advance
* don't nag or complain
* separate the smoking from from the smoker - focus on the behavior
* let your friend(s) know how you feel about smoking in your house, car, etc. - be courteous

Quitting
Page #387

List five things you can do to help your friend Maura quit smoking.
1. _____
2. _____
3. _____
4. _____
5. _____

15/40

* each day, have your first cigarette 15 minutes later than yesterday
* distract yourself when you crave tobacco
* establish, then extend, nonsmoking hours
* if you smoke after eating, then do something else
* never smoke two packs of the same brand in a row
* buy by the pack, not the carton
* make it harder to get at your cigarettes (lock them up)
* smoke with the hand you don't normally use
* smoke only half of each cigarette
* keep daily records of tobacco use
* don't empty ashtrays

Quitting
Page #388

What are seven techniques for cutting down on the number of cigarettes you smoke?

1. _____
2. _____
3. _____
4. _____
5. _____
6. _____
7. _____

15/41

1) identify your smoking habits - keep a diary
2) get support from a friend
3) begin by tapering off - cut down for 1-4 weeks
4) set a quit date - make a big event out of your announcement
5) stop - smoke only 5/day the week before you quit; smoke them in the evening in close succession
6) follow-up - keep in touch with your support system during the first few weeks; remind yourself that you're becoming a better person each day

Quitting
Page #391

Outline a six-point program for quitting smoking.

1. _____
2. _____
3. _____
4. _____
5. _____
6. _____

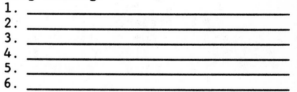

Essay

15/42   The export of American tobacco products is now being considered more
         seriously by a federal administration concerned about our trade
         deficit. As concerns about the health risks associated with tobacco
         use continue to depress the domestic tobacco market, cigarette
         manufacturers have turned their marketing energies toward the
         international marketplace in general, and the Third World in
         particular. Needless to say, the warnings we are used to seeing on
         cigarette packaging are not printed on most cigarette packs sold
         outside the U.S. What responsibilities, if any, do you believe
         domestic tobacco companies have with regard to the health risks their
         products pose to foreign consumers? Defend your answer.

15/43   Many rural families depend on tobacco for their economic livelihood.
         For many tobacco farmers, the federal tobacco subsidy program provides
         a safety net against falling prices. Critics contend that this
         program maintains and extends the dependence that these families have
         on a crop which has, at best, a limited future. What do you think is
         going to happen to tobacco farmers in the U.S., and how (if at all)
         should federal and state governments assist tobacco farmers?

15/44   Passive smoking continues to be a topic of controversy. Most often,
         discussions focus on the "rights of nonsmokers to breathe clean air"
         vs. the "rights of smokers to smoke." Are there other issues that
         need to be included in this discussion? If so, what are they? If
         not, where do you see the rights of smokers ending and the rights of
         nonsmokers begining?

15/45   For years, families of those who have died of lung cancer or emphysema
         have brought legal action against cigarette companies. Most often,
         these suits claim that the manufacturer should bear some, if not all,
         of the responsibility for making, promoting, and selling a dangerous
         product. The standard response is that smoking is a personal
         decision, and the individual must bear the consequences. Do you think
         it's ethical to manufacture, promote, and sell an addictive substance?
         If so, should access to this substance be regulated? How? If it's
         not ethical, do you think our legal system provides sufficient
         protection for the consumer? If yes, how? If not, why not?

AN INVITATION TO HEALTH
TEST BANK

Section V - Understanding Your Risks

Chapter 16: Consumer Health

In this chapter -

* Self-Care
* Practitioners
* Preventive Care
* Responsible Consumerism
* Health-Care Costs
* Quackery

Section V - Understanding Your Risks
Chapter 16: Consumer Health

True-False

16/1	False Self-Care Page #399	Recent trends in health care have re- sulted in increased emphasis on the diseased part of the patient.
16/2	True Self-Care Page #400	Vital signs are basic physiological measurements taken in order to assess one's state of health.
16/3	True Self-Care Page #400	A blood pressure reading of 120/80 would be considered within the normal range for most adults.
16/4	False Self-Care Page #400	Commercially available cold medica- tions can be effectively used to cure a cold.
16/5	True Self-Care Page #402	It is possible to become physically and psychologically dependent on over-the-counter drugs.
16/6	False Practitioners Page #403	Physicians comprise about 25% of all health-care practitioners.
16/7	True Practitioners Page #405	Primary care physicians, or family practitioners, are the primary link between patients and medical special- ists.
16/8	True Preventive Care Page #410	Most physicians now believe that com- plete physical examinations need not be performed annually for young and middle aged persons who feel well.
16/9	True Preventive Care Page #411	Mild hypertension is indicated by a blood pressure reading of 140/90 or higher.
16/10	False Responsible Consumerism Page #413	Patient histories are not critical to effective diagnosis and treatment.
16/11	True Responsible Consumerism Page #413	Compliance is a term used to describe the degree to which a patient follows through on the recommendations of a physician.

16/12   False
Responsible Consumerism
Page #415

Discussions between the physician and patient regarding precautions and side effects of a <u>new</u> drug prescription occur in the majority of cases.

16/13   True
Responsible Consumerism
Page #415

The generic name of a drug is really its chemical name.

16/14   True
Responsible Consumerism
Page #416

Unnecessary surgery is a significant health care problem in the U.S.

16/15   False
Responsible Consumerism
Page #419

Physicians are required by law to guarantee good results to their patients.

16/16   True
Health-Care Costs
Page #419

Health care in the U.S. costs more than $1 billion per day.

16/17   True
Health-Care Costs
Page #421

Members of health maintenance organizations (HMO's) spend 65% less time in hospitals than the national average.

16/18   False
Health-Care Costs
Page #423

The introduction of Medicare reimbursement based on diagnosis-related groups, or DRG's, has resulted in longer stays in the hospital for many patients.

16/19   True
Alternatives
Page #423

"Holistic" alternatives to traditional medicine emphasize the importance of treating the complete person, not just the illness.

16/20   True
Quackery
Page #424

Each year, Americans spend about $10 billion on unproven health products and services.

Multiple Choice

16/21   a
Self-Care
Page #400

Your vital signs include temperature, blood pressure, pulse rate, and

a. respiration rate.
b. weight.
c. cholesterol level.
d. basal metabolism rate.

16/22   b
         Self-Care
         Page #402

Acetaminophen (Tylenol, Tempra, etc.)
is effective for all of the following
except

a. controlling fever.
b. reducing inflammation.
c. relieving pain.
d. avoiding stomach upset associated
   with aspirin use.

16/23   d
         Self-Care
         Page #402

The most commonly abused over-the-
counter drugs include nasal sprays,
laxatives, and

a. children's cold medications.
b. aspirin.
c. hemorrhoid medications.
d. eye drops.

16/24   d
         Practitioners
         Pages #403-404

Registered nurses

a. are supervised by licensed, practical nurses.
b. today are not required to earn a
   bachelor's degree.
c. supervise nurse practitioners.
d. must graduate from a school of
   nursing approved by a state board.

16/25   c
         Practitioners
         Page #404

Medical specialization

a. training can be substituted for
   the 1 year hospital internship required for most doctors.
b. training includes a 1 year residency
   in addition to the internship.
c. is usually organized around specific
   diseases or organ systems.
d. does not require certification.

16/26   b
         Preventive Care
         Page #410

Kaiser-Permanente, a health maintenance
organization, recommends that an individual between the ages of 18 and 35
years have a complete checkup every

a. 5 years.
b. 4 years.
c. 3 years
d. 2 years.

16/27   a
Preventive Care
Page #411

The most important health screening tests include blood-pressure readings, Pap smears, tuberculosis and glaucoma tests, and

a. breast examinations.
b. body temperature.
c. height and weight measurement.
d. electrocardiogram.

16/28   c
Preventive Care
Page #411

Pap smears are used to detect

a. breast cancer.
b. tuberculosis.
c. cervical cancer.
d. glaucoma.

16/29   d
Responsible Consumerism
Page #413

Which of the following statements about prescription drugs is most accurate?

a. Pharmacists have exclusive authority to dispense prescription drugs.
b. Physicians have exclusive authority to prescribe drugs.
c. In order to become a drug that can be prescribed by a physician, the drug must be proved effective.
d. The majority of prescription drugs now available do not have proven effectiveness according to the FDA.

16/30   b
Responsible Consumerism
Page #415

Generic drugs

a. are chemically different from their brand name counterparts, but have nearly the same effect.
b. are not always less expensive than brand names equivalents.
c. use identical fillers and binders during their manufacture.
d. are more effective than brand names for the treatment of heart disease and seizure disorders (epilepsy).

16/31   a
Responsible Consumerism
Page #417

Outpatient surgical centers

a. can be up to 50% less expensive than standard hospital fees.
b. handle routine emergency treatment.
c. have higher complication rates than hospitals.
d. are set up to provide extended, postoperative care.

16/32   d
         Responsible Consumerism
         Page #417

Advantages to home health care include all of the following except

a. reduced costs.
b. convenience.
c. use of advanced technology.
d. complete health insurance coverage.

16/33   c
         Responsible Consumerism
         Page #419

The most common basis for malpractice lawsuits is

a. failure to obtain consent for an operation.
b. compromise of a patient's confidentiality.
c. failure to provide service with appropriate knowledge and skill.
d. failure to inform the patient of critical information.

16/34   b
         Health-Care Costs
         Page #420

Which of the following statements about medical care payment methods is most accurate?

a. Method of payment has been shown to affect the quality of medical care the patient receives.
b. Prepaid systems usually result in a 20% savings over fee-for-service systems.
c. Fee-for-service systems effectively remove the profit motive from medical care.
d. Fee-for-service systems usually cost the patient about 20% less than prepaid systems.

16/35   c
         Health-Care Costs
         Page #420

All of the following are available health insurance options except

a. Medicare, which pays 80% of most medical bills for people over age 65.
b. Medicaid, which uses state and federal funds to provide coverage for people who can't afford insurance.
c. supplemental health insurance, which provides total health insurance coverage.
d. major-medical policies, designed to cover routine doctor and hospital expenses.

16/36   d
Health-Care Costs
Page #422

Which of the following is not a type of health maintenance organization?

a. Closed-panel HMO
b. Independent Practice Association, or IPA
c. Preferred-provider Organization, or PPO
d. Diagnosis-related Group, or DRG

16/37   b
Alternatives
Page #422

Which of the following is not a factor contributing to falling levels of satisfaction with conventional medicine?

a. growing concern about the dangers of prescription drugs
b. fears that modern technology is under-utilized in favor of person-to-person treatment
c. resentment of high medical bills
d. growing interest in preventive medicine and self-care

16/38   a
Quackery
Page #424

The appeal of quackery depends on

a. the level of suffering and desperation of the victim(s).
b. the medical value of the quack's product or service.
c. the price of the product or service.
d. the lack of information about safe alternatives.

Completion

16/39   * talk to your friends; get specific details about the treatment they receive
* call the nearest teaching hospital and get a list of staff and affiliated physicians
* find out which hospital your doctor or dentist admits to: if it's a teaching hospital, find out what that means should you be admitted
* call their secretary and find out about their medical credentials
* find out if they are in a solo or group practice
Practitioners
Page #406

What are four things you can do to find a competent physician or dentist you will be comfortable with.
1.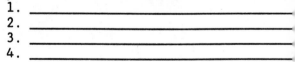
2. _____
3. _____
4. _____

16/40   Does your doctor -
          * explain procedures to you?
          * encourage you to ask ques-
            tions?
          * give you straight answers?
          * listen to your problems?
          * provide reassurance when
            you're concerned?
          * spend enough time with
            you?
          * take thorough histories?
          * prescribe drugs for every
            patient?
          * recommend expensive ser-
            vices too enthusiastically?
          * admit to not having all the
            answers and make referrals
            when necessary?
          Practitioners
          Page #407

Your friend has been complaining to
you about her doctor. List six questions you could ask her to help clear
up her concerns.
1. _____
2. _____
3. _____
4. _____
5. _____
6. _____

16/41   * specifically why the test
            is needed
          * could earlier test results
            be used instead
          * what are the risks of
            waiting and not testing
          * what about false positives
            and negatives; what hap-
            pens if the test is posi-
            tive
          * what are the risks invol-
            ved with the procedure
          * effect of allergies or
            medicine you are taking
          * how long will the test take
            and how do you prepare for
            it
          Preventive Care
          Page #412

Your physician has recommended a test
for you, and you're not sure you should
comply. State five areas to explore
before going along with the procedure.
1. _____
2. _____
3. _____
4. _____
5. _____

16/42   * the name of the drug
          * what it is supposed to do
          * how and when it is taken
          * how long it is taken
          * what foods, drinks, or ac-
            tivities should be avoid-
            ed while taking the drug
          * what the side effects are
            and what to do if they oc-
            cur
          * is there written informa-
            tion available for the drug
          Responsible Consumerism
          Page #415

What are four things you should know
about a prescription drug before taking
it?
1. _____
2. _____
3. _____
4. _____

16/43   * What will happen if I
       don't get the surgery?
* How long can I delay in
   order to try other treat-
   ments?
* What are the risks and
   side effects?
* Do the risks change if I
   delay surgery?
* Are there nonsurgical treat-
   ments available? What
   are their side effects?
* Could I live comfortably
   without surgery? How long?
* Can I talk with those who
   have had the procedure?
   Those who declined?
* What are the details of
   the actual procedure?
Responsible Consumerism
Page #416

Identify six questions to ask before
going ahead with surgery.
1. _____
2. _____
3. _____
4. _____
5. _____
6. _____

16/44   * are there provisions that
       cover loss of income
* what costs are covered by
   the insurance
* what family members are
   covered
* is there convalescent-care
   coverage
* is there extended-care
   coverage
* what the maximum benefits
   are
* what the waiting periods
   and exclusions are
* what the deductibles and
   coinsurance provisions are
* who has renewal rights
Costs
Page #421

Name five things to ask about health
insurance.
1. _____
2. _____
3. _____
4. _____

Matching

16/45   Directions: Match each of the common ailments listed on the left with the correct treatment on the right. Each treatment **may** be used only once.

	Ailment	Treatment
1.	__ Congestion	a. methylcellulose drops
2.	__ Coughs	b. clear liquid diet, Kaopectate
3.	__ Constipation	c. pseudoephedrine (Sudafed)
4.	__ Diarrhea	d. penicillin
5.	__ Eye Irritations	e. nonabsorbable antacids
6.	__ Hemorrhoids	f. Ipecac syrup
7.	__ Pain and Fever	g. Castor oil
8.	__ Poisoning (<u>not</u> petro- leum-based or strong acid/alkali)	h. zinc oxide creams i. high-fiber diet j. aspirin/acetaminophen
9.	__ Upset Stomach	k. expectorants (glyceryl guaiacolate)

1-c, 2-k, 3-i, 4-b, 5-a,
6-h, 7-j, 8-f, 9-e
Self-Care

16/46   Directions: Match each of the medical specialties on the left with its correct description on the right. Each description may be used only once.

	Specialty	Description
1.	__ Clinical Psychologists	a. deal with foot problems
2.	__ Optometrists	b. use bone manipulation to relieve nervous system strain/tension
3.	__ Ophthalmologists	c. provide mental health services
4.	__ Podiatrists	d. diagnose vision problems and pre- scribe glasses
5.	__ Chiropractors	e. diseases and treatment of children
		f. diagnose eye diseases, perform surgery on the eye(s)

1-c, 2-d, 3-f, 4-a, 5-b
Practitioners
Pages #403-406

Essay

16/47   In your lifetime, you will probably know someone who has AIDS. What would you say to this person if they were to tell you that they were considering a radical, new form of treatment not yet available in the U.S.?

16/48   California has recently imposed some limits on the amount of damages that can be awarded for malpractice judgements. Do you think there should be financial limits to a physician's liability? If yes, why? not, who should bear the expense of huge insurance settlements?

16/49   Do you think physicians should be allowed to advertise their charges, and promote their services like any other business? Why, or why not?

16/50   A number of countries have adopted a socialized approach to medicine, where the government has primary responsibility for providing medical care. What do you see as the advantages and disadvantages to the consumer of this type of arrangement?

Section V - Understanding Your Risks

Chapter 17: Cardiovascular Health

In this chapter -

* Risk Factors
* Cardiovascular Disease
* Treatment
* Stroke

Section V - Understanding Your Risks
Chapter 17: Cardiovascular Health

True-False

17/1   True   Heart disease accounts for almost 50%
         Risk Factors   of all deaths in the U.S.
         Page #429

17/2   True   Over the past 10 years, the death rate
         Risk Factors   from heart disease has fallen 25%.
         Page #429

17/3   False   Heredity is the most important factor
         Risk Factors   in assessing the risk of cardiovacular
         Page #430   disease.

17/4   True   Smoking is the most dangerous risk
         Risk Factors   factor for heart disease.
         Page #431

17/5   False   The symptoms of high blood pressure
         Risk Factors   include chest pain, dizziness, and
         Page #432   fatigue.

17/6   True   A 1 percent drop in blood cholesterol
         Risk Factors   level results in a 2 percent reduction
         Page #433   in heart-attack risk.

17/7   True   The cause of hypertension is unknown in
         Risk Factors   the majority of cases.
         Page #438

17/8   False   Successful management of hypertension
         Risk Factors   does not require patient compliance.
         Page #438

17/9   False   Angina pectoris is a pain in the chest
         Cardiovascular Disease   that signals the beginning of a heart
         Page #439   attack.

17/10   True   A myocardial infarction occurs when a
         Cardiovascular Disease   portion of heart muscle dies due to
         Pages #439-440   lack of oxygen.

17/11   False   Heart tissue affected during a heart
         Cardiovascular Disease   attack is immediately and permanently
         Page #442   destroyed.

17/12   True
         Cardiovascular Disase   Most people who have a heart attack re-
         Page #442   turn to productive lives after 2 to 3
                                        months of recuperation.

17/13   True
         Cardiovascular Disease   An aspirin every other day has been
         Page #441   shown to prevent heart attacks in
                                        healthy men.

17/14   True
         Cardiovascular Disease   An arrhythmia is an irregular heart-
         Page #442   beat.

17/15   False
         Treatment   The electrocardiogram (EKG) is the most
         Page #443   complete and accurate diagnostic test
                                        for the heart.

17/16   True
         Treatment   Most people with heart disease can be
         Page #444   successfully treated with drugs.

17/17   False
         Treatment   Coronary bypass operations have been
         Page #444   shown to be significantly more effec-
                                        tive than medical treatment alone in
                                        treating all forms of artery block-
                                        age.

17/18   True
         Treatment   80% of all heart transplant recipients
         Page #446   are alive after 1 year.

17/19   True
         Stroke   A stroke is caused by an interruption
         Page #447   of the blood supply to the brain.

17/20   True
         Stroke   Brain cells injured during a stroke
         Page #447   cannot regenerate themselves.

Multiple Choice

17/21   d
         Risk Factors   X   Cardiovascular disease is caused by all
         Page #430   of the following except

                                        a. the flow of blood to the heart is
                                           blocked.
                                        b. the flow of blood through the heart
                                           to the body is blocked.
                                        c. a malfunction in the specialized
                                           cells that generate electical im-
                                           pulses and coordinate contractions.
                                        d. cardiac arrhythmias, or irregulari-
                                           ties in the heart rate.

17/22   c
           Risk Factors
           Page #431

Which of the following statements about risk factors for heart disease is most accurate?

a. Cardiovascular disease can be inherited.
b. The incidence of hypertension among Black Americans places this group at a somewhat lower risk for heart disease than their Caucasian peers.
c. The rate of deaths from heart attacks increases with age.
d. Working women have a higher rate of heart problems than those who stay at home.

17/23   a
           Risk Factors
           Page #431

The **least** likely explanation for how cigarettes damage the heart is

a. the tar in cigarettes causes clots in the blood.
b. the nicotine in cigarettes overstimulating the heart.
c. by the displacement of oxygen in the blood by carbon monoxide in cigarette smoke.
d. the smoke damages the lining of the arteries, thus encouraging the buildup of cholesterol.

17/24   b
           Risk Factors
           Page #432

The relationship between lipoproteins and heart health is best described by which statement?

a. Low-density lipoproteins (LDLs) are desirable because they reduce the density of cholesterol in the blood.
b. The higher the ratio of high-density lipoproteins (HDL) to total cholesterol, the lower the likelihood of heart disease.
c. Lowering high-density lipoprotein levels reduces the risk of heart attacks.
d. Women are much more likely to develop heart problems before menopause.

17/25   c
Risk Factors
Page #433

The presence of cholesterol in the bloodstream is important with regard to heart disease because

a. 50% of all Americans have danger-ously high levels.
b. high cholesterol levels cannot be treated.
c. it is a reliable indicator of the buildup of plaque on the inner walls of arteries.
d. high levels of cholesterol mean you have heart disease.

17/26   c
Risk Factors
Page #433

According to the National Heart, Lung and Blood Institute (NHLBI), it is neither normal nor healthy to have a cholesterol level above

a. 150 mg/dl.
b. 175 mg/dl.
c. 200 mg/dl.
d. 225 mg/dl.

17/27   d
Risk Factors
Page #434

Heart specialists describe a low-fat diet as one which derives no more than

a. 50% of its calories from fat in any form, and not more than 25% from saturated fat.
b. 40% of its calories from all forms of fat.
c. 20% of its calories from saturated fat.
d. 30% of its calories from fat in any form, and not more than 10% from saturated fat.

17/28   a
Cardiovascular Disease
Page #438

The impact of hypertension on the heart is to

a. cause enlargement of the left side from the excess work load.
b. cause arrhythmias because of the in-creased work load.
c. weaken the heart muscle as a result of muscle stress.
d. reduce the actual amount of blood in the body.

17/29   c
Cardiovascular Disease
Page #438

A blood pressure reading of 145/95 in a young adult would be considered

a. below normal.
b. normal.
c. borderline hypertensive.
d. definite hypertensive.

17/30   d
Cardiovascular Disease
Page #438

Each of the following comments about atherosclerosis is true except

a. it is the most common form of arter-iosclerosis.
b. it may begin in childhood.
c. it is the underlying cause of most heart attacks.
d. it has not been shown to be related to the buildup of plaque in the arteries.

17/31   b
Cardiovascular Disease
Page #439

Coronary artery spasms may be triggered by smoking, stress, clumping of platelets in the bloodstream, and

a. a diet deficient in calcium.
b. the presence of excess calcium in smooth muscle cells.
c. blockages in the arteries.
d. angina.

17/32   a
Cardiovascular Disease
Page #440

Which of the following statements about heart attacks is most accurate?

a. They are _caused_ by an interruption of oxygen and nutrients to heart muscle.
b. They _result_ in an interruption of oxygen and nutrients to the heart.
c. Most people with heart attack symptoms seek help within the first critical hour.
d. Most people who die of a heart attack do so in the hospital.

17/33   c
Cardiovascular Disease
Page #441

Streptokinase, aspirin, and t-PA are all

a. used to treat arrhythmias.
b. used to treat angina.
c. drugs effective in dissolving clots.
d. remedies that have been proven ineffective in treating heart disease.

17/34   b
Cardiovascular Disease
Page #442

Following a heart attack,

a. most people require at least one year of recuperation before returning to an active life.
b. new blood vessels are formed to take blood through the area of damaged tissue.
c. the affected area can rarely be healed.
d. collateral circulation is no longer possible.

17/35   d
Cardiovascular Disease
Page #442

Congestive heart failure is characterized primarily by

a. angina.
b. cyanosis.
c. a buildup of fluids in the heart muscle.
d. an accumulation of blood fluids in the body's extremities and lungs.

17/36   a
Treatment
Page #444

Which of the following statements about coronary bypass operations is most accurate?

a. It is more effective than medical treatment alone in prolonging life in certain patients with specific problems.
b. It is more effective than medical treatment in prolonging life for all types of heart disease.
c. Less than 50% of all bypass patients develop blockages in the grafted vessel(s) within 10 years.
d. It is a procedure that involves rerouting a blood vessel from one of the heart to another.

17/37   c
Treatment
Page #444

Percutaneous Transluminal Coronary Angioplasty (PTCA), or balloon angioplasty,

a. is only successful in about 30%-40% of all patients undergoing the procedure.
b. is generally riskier than heart bypass surgery.
c. is an effective form of treatment during and following a heart attack.
d. involves grafting a vein from the leg onto the diseased area of the heart.

17/38   a
Treatment
Page #446

With regard to heart transplants,

a. more than 80% of all heart recipients are alive after 1 year.
b. less than half live longer than 5 years.
c. donors outnumber potential recipients.
d. of all survivors, only a small percentage are in good health.

17/39   d
Stroke
Page #447

Strokes, or cerebrovascular accidents,

a. kill more people each year than cancer or heart disease.
b. always result in permanent loss of physical or mental functions.
c. kill over half the people who have one.
d. require strong preventive measures since injured brain cells cannot regenerate themselves like other organs.

17/40   c
Stroke
Page #447

People at highest risk for a stroke are

a. those who have low red blood cell counts.
b. white females.
c. those who have experienced a transient ischemic attack (TIA).
d. those who abuse aspirin.

Completion

17/41   * go to your physician or health department to have your cholesterol level checked
* ask about the accuracy of the test/instrument
* think about timing your checkup to coincide with a routine physical exam
* let you doctor know if you are taking drugs
* follow recommended procedures exactly
* get "real" numbers, not just "high" or "low"
* get your HDL/LDL ratio
Risk Factors
Page #433

Being tested for cholesterol has become more convenient, although not every testing site is the same. Name 4 things to consider if you plan to have your cholesterol level checked.
1. _____
2. _____
3. _____
4. _____

17/42
* a heavy squeezing or discomfort in the center of the chest
* a pain radiating to the shoulder, arm, jaw or neck
* anxiety
* sweating
* nausea and vomiting
* shortness of breath
* dizziness or fainting
Cardiovascular Disease
Page #440

Identify five warning signals of a heart attack.
1. _____
2. _____
3. _____
4. _____
5. _____

17/43
* call the emergency rescue service, or go the nearest hospital with emergency cardiac care
* give cardiopulmonary resuscitation (CPR) if you are trained and if it is necessary
Cardiovascular Disease
Page #442

If you are with someone who has the "signals" of a heart attack for more than 2 minutes, what are the 2 most important things to do?
1. _____
2. _____

17/44
* sudden weakness/numbness of face, arm, or leg
* temporary loss of speech, difficulty in speaking/understanding
* double vision
* unexplained dizziness
* change in personality
* change in pattern of headaches
Stroke
Page #447

What are four warning signs of a stroke?
1. _____
2. _____
3. _____
4. _____

17/45
* don't smoke
* maintain proper body weight
* eat foods low in fat and cholesterol
* get regular exercise
* if you use oral contraceptives, get regular checkups
* manage your response to stress effectively
Risk Factors
Pages #430-435

What are four things you can do to have a healthy heart.
1. _____
2. _____
3. _____
4. _____

<u>Matching</u>

17/46   Directions: Match each of the terms on the left with its correct
         definition on the right. Each definition may be used only once.

              <u>Term</u>   <u>Definition</u>
         1. __ arteriosclerosis   a. pain or discomfort in the chest
         2. __ atherosclerosis   b. a blockage in an artery
         3. __ plaque   c. any impairment of blood flow
         4. __ thrombosis   through the arteries
         5. __ angina pectoris   d. a cerebrovascular accident
         6. __ platelet   e. a disease of the arteries marked by
                                           formation of plaque on the inner
                                           walls
                                        f. fragments of a blood cell that
                                           assist in clotting
                                        g. deposits of fat and other materials
                                           on the wall of an artery

         1-c, 2-e, 3-g,
         4-b, 5-a, 6-f
         Cardiovascular Disease
         Pages #433-448

17/47   Directions: Match each of the terms on the left with its correct
         definition on the right. Each definition may be used only once.

              <u>Term</u>   <u>Definition</u>
         1. __ collateral circulation a. a heart rate less than 60 beats per
         2. __ tachycardia   minute
         3. __ bradycardia   b. formation of new blood vessels
         4. __ atrial fibrillation   c. irregular heartbeat
         5. __ arrhythmia   d. insufficient oxygen in the blood
         6. __ cyanosis   e. heart attack
                                        f. a heart rate over 100 beats per
                                           minute
                                        g. diffusion of electrical impulses
                                           throughout the heart

         1-b, 2-f, 3-a
         4-g, 5-c, 6-d
         Cardiovascular Disease
         Pages #430-448

Chapter 17: Cardiovascular Disease

Essay

17/48   With limited resources available to meet expanding health care
needs, many new, experimental procedures such as artificial heart
implantation are being criticized because they are so expensive.
Critics argue that health care resources should be allocated to meet
the basic needs of all people before dollars are spent on
extraordinary situations such as heart transplants. Do you believe
that access to medical care should be determined by one's ability to
pay? If not, what criteria should be used?

     If you had $1 million to spend on health care, and had to choose
between a single, life saving operation for one person that was
highly experimental, or an array of **preventive** services and
treatments for a number of people, which would you choose? Defend
the criteria you used to arrive at your answer.

17/49   While advances in treatment have been effective in reducing the toll
of heart disease in our society, aspects of our lifestyle (diet,
smoking, etc.) continue to put us at risk. Oftentimes, changes in
behavior have been successfully brought about through legislation.
If you could pass one law directed at reducing the risk of heart
disease for the general population, what would it be? Defend your
answer.

17/50   Every person is at risk, to some degree, for heart disease. Based
on what you know about risk factors, describe your own personal
level of risk for acquiring heart disease. What factors did you
take into account? What options, if any, do you have for reducing
your level of risk?

AN INVITATION TO HEALTH
TEST BANK

Section V - Understanding Your Risks

Chapter 18: Cancer, Major Illnesses,
                  and Accidents

In this chapter -

*   Cancer
*   Prevention
*   Types
*   Diagnosis/Therapy
*   Major Illnesses
*   Accidents

Section V - Understanding Your Risks
Chapter 18: Cancer, Major Illnesses, and Accidents

True-False

18/1   True
        Cancer
        Page #451

Cancer kills one out of every five
Americans.

18/2   True
        Cancer
        Page #451

About half of all patients diagnosed
with cancer survive for at least
five years after the diagnosis.

18/3   False
        Cancer
        Page #451

Cancer is a single disease that appears
at different sites throughout the body.

18/4   True
        Cancer
        Page #453

The higher death rate from cancer among
Blacks is due to socioeconomic, not
racial, factors.

18/5   False
        Cancer
        Page #454

Diet does not play a role in causing
cancer.

18/6   True
        Prevention
        Page #455

The rates for people getting cancer, as
well as the rates for people dying from
cancer, rose between 1975 and 1981.

18/7   True
        Types
        Page #456

Heavy cigarette smokers account for as
much as 90% of all lung cancer cases
diagnosed each year.

18/8   False
        Types
        Page #460

The rate of cervical cancer is rising
steadily.

18/9   False
        Types
        Page #460

Cancers of the colon and rectum are
relatively rare compared to leukemia
or oral cancer.

18/10   True
        Types
        Page #461

The most common form of cancer is skin
cancer.

18/11   False
        Types
        Page #462

Leukemia stikes more children than
adults.

18/12	True Diagnosis/Therapy Page #467	Early diagnosis of cancer signifi-cantly improves one's chances of survival.
18/13	True Diagnosis/Therapy Page #467	Former cancer patients are protected from discrimination by federal laws that protect the handicapped.
18/14	False Major Illnesses Page #467	Most diabetics require daily injections of insulin in order to survive.
18/15	True Major Illnesses Page #469	Anemias are diseases of the blood that reduce its oxygen-carrying capacity.
18/16	False Major Illnesses Page #469	Epilepsy is frequently fatal.
18/17	False Major Illnesses Page #470	Cirrhosis is an early sign of liver damage.
18/18	True Major Illnesses Page #472	Most arthritis victims below the age of 70 are women.
18/19	False Major Illnesses Page #472	Hernias occur only in the groin area.
18/20	True Accidents Page #473	For persons between the ages of 15 and 24, accidents are responsible for more deaths than all other causes combined.

Multiple Choice

18/21	b Cancer Page #452	Cells from a cancerous tumor differ from those in a benign tumor because they divide more often, vary more in shape and size than normal cells, and

a. have smaller nuclei.
b. have larger nuclei.
c. have no nuclei at all.
d. attack normal cells.

18/22   a
Cancer
Page #452

Which of the following statements about cancer causes is <u>least</u> accurate?

a. Most cancers have a single cause.
b. Cancer causing chemicals are a natural part of our daily diet.
c. Tanning machines are just as dangerous as natural sunlight in their effect on the skin.
d. Heredity may make certain families cancer-prone.

18/23   d
Cancer
Page #454

Which of the following statements most accurately describes the relationship between diet and cancer?

a. Diet affects a higher percentage of cancers in men than women.
b. Fatty foods reduce the risk of certain types of cancer.
c. Vitamin intake doesn't really affect your risk of contracting cancer.
d. Obesity and cured foods increase the risks of cancer.

18/24   c
Prevention
Page #456

Which of the following is <u>not</u> a screening test for cancer?

a. mammogram
b. pap test
c. mastectomy
d. stool blood test

18/25   c
Types
Page #456

Which of the following statements about lung cancer is most accurate?

a. The early stages of lung cancer can be detected quite easily.
b. Lung cancer has one of the highest 5 year survival rates among all cancers.
c. Quitting smoking for 10 years reduces one's risk for lung cancer to nearly the level of someone who has never smoked.
d. Chest pain is not a symptom of lung cancer.

18/26   a   All of the following are true with re-
           Types   gard to breast cancer except:
           Page #458
                                 a. The radical mastectomy is the most
                                    effective form of surgical treat-
                                    ment for breast cancer.
                                 b. Changes in the appearance, feel,
                                    or function of the breast are pri-
                                    mary warning signals for breast
                                    cancer.
                                 c. Mammograms are a recommended form
                                    of early detection for women aged
                                    35 and over.
                                 d. For breast cancer that has not
                                    spread at all, the five year sur-
                                    vival rate is nearly 100%.

18/27   d   Cervical cancer
           Types
           Page #460   a. rates have increased steadily over
                                    the past 10 years.
                                 b. occurs most frequently in women of
                                    higher socioeconomic status.
                                 c. is treated primarily with chemo-
                                    therapy.
                                 d. risk factors include early age of
                                    first intercourse, multiple sex
                                    partners, and a history of genital
                                    herpes.

18/28   b   Colon and rectum cancers
           Types
           Page #461   a. usually result in a colostomy, or
                                    permanent abdominal opening for the
                                    elimination of wastes.
                                 b. can cause unusual bleeding from the
                                    rectum, blood in the stool, or
                                    changes in bowel habits.
                                 c. are unrelated to a family history
                                    of similar problems.
                                 d. are not related to dietary patterns.

18/29   d   With regard to cancers that affect men,
           Types
           Page #463   a. testicular cancer is most common in
                                    men over the age of 35.
                                 b. prostate cancer is most common in
                                    men under age 35.
                                 c. symptoms of a prostate problem
                                    usually indicate the presence of
                                    cancer.
                                 d. testicular self-examinations are an
                                    easy and effective method for early
                                    detection of testicular cancer.

18/30   b
Diagnosis Therapy
Page #464

Which of the following statements about cancer therapy is most accurate?

a. Radiation therapy affects only the malignant cells in the body.
b. Combinations of treatements often provide the best therapeutic results.
c. Radiation and chemotherapy are most effective against slower-growing cells in the body.
d. Surgery is responsible for only a small percentage of cancer cures each year.

18/31   a
Diagnosis/Therapy
Page #464

The form of radiation therapy that involves placing radioactive material directly into a malignancy is called

a. interstitial implantation.
b. interstitial hyperthermia.
c. particle therapy.
d. radioactive-labeled antibodies.

18/32   d
Diagnosis/Therapy
Page #467

All of the following are associated with recovery from cancer except

a. reduced health benefits.
b. on-the-job discrimination.
c. work as an effective psychological therapy.
d. expanded life insurance coverage.

18/33   b
Major Illnesses
Page #467

Which of the following statements about diabetes mellitus is most accurate?

a. More people die from diabetes itself than from associated complications such as kidney disease or stroke.
b. The complications associated with diabetes kill far more people than the disease itself.
c. Diabetes is a rare disorder.
d. Diabetes is caused by overproduction of insulin by the pancreas.

18/34   a
         Major Illnesses
         Page #467

With regard to diabetes mellitus,

a. the most common symptoms include
   frequent urination and excessive
   thirst.
b. over 75% of those with the disease
   are diagnosed before the age of 25.
c. less than one half of all complications which arise from it are
   preventable or treatable.
d. the majority of people in the
   United States who have it are
   dependent on insulin.

18/35   c
         Major Illnesses
         Page #469

Which of the following is <u>least</u> likely
to trigger an attack in an asthma-
prone person?

a. respiratory infection
b. stress
c. change in diet habits
d. allergy

18/36   b
         Major Illnesses
         Page #469

Which of the following factors do <u>all</u>
anemias have in common?

a. insufficient vitamin B in the diet
b. reduced oxygen-carrying capacity of
   the blood
c. crescent-shaped hemoglobin
d. insufficient dietary iron

18/37   c
         Major Illnesses
         Page #470

Each of the following statements about
epilepsy is true except one:

a. The severity of epilepsy is defined
   by the frequency of attacks.
b. Most epileptics have grand mal
   seizures.
c. Less than 25% of all cases of epilepsy are of unknown origin.
d. Petit mal seizures are marked by
   random movement and/or unintelli-
   gible sounds.

18/38   a
         Major Illnesses
         Page #470

Chronic kidney damage, or nephrosis,
is characterized by

a. high levels of fats in the blood.
b. loss of water/fluid from body
   tissue.
c. increased protein in the urine.
d. kidney stones.

18/39   c
         Major Illnesses
         Page #471

Which of the following digestive disorders is most life-threatening?

a. ulcers
b. gallstones
c. Crohn's disease
d. irritable bowel syndrome

18/40   d
         Major Illnesses
         Page #472

All of the following are true of
arthritis, except

a. it becomes more common and severe
   with age.
b. women are generally affected more
   often than men.
c. rheumatoid arthritis is fairly
   common among younger people.
d. 50% of all Americans over the age
   of 65 are affected by some form of
   arthritis.

18/41   a
         Accidents
         Page #473

Automobile and motorcycle accidents

a. are the primary cause of accidental
   death in the U.S.
b. are rarely fatal and/or serious at
   speeds of less than 40 m.p.h.
c. that result in fatalities usually
   occur on long-distance trips, far
   away from home.
d. are usually due to bad luck.

18/42   d
         Accidents
         Page #475

With regard to common accidents,

a. deaths caused by falls in the home
   are quite rare.
b. most victims of accidental poisoning are over the age of 5 years.
c. hypothermia occurs most frequently
   in temperatures below the freezing
   point.
d. most victims of drowning are teen-
   age boys.

Completion

18/43   * cigarette smoking
         Cancer
         Page #453

What is the single most significant
cause of cancer in the U.S. today?

_____

18/44
* cut fat intake to 30%
  of total calories
* increase fiber intake
* include calcium in
  in your daily diet
* eat fish 2 or 3 times
  each week
* eat two or three vege-
  tables per day
* choose foods rich in
  vitamins A, C, and E
* limit your intake of
  salt-cured, smoked &
  pickled foods
Prevention
Page #454

Identify four diet-related changes you
can make to reduce your risk of cancer.
1. _____
2. _____
3. _____
4. _____

18/45
* a change in bowel or
  bladder habits
* a sore that doesn't
  heal
* unusual bleeding or
  discharge
* a thickening or lump
  (especially in the
  breast)
* indigestion or dif-
  ficulty swallowing
* an obvious change in
  a wart or mole
* a nagging cough or
  hoarseness
Prevention
Page #456

Name the seven warning signs of cancer.
1. _____
2. _____
3. _____
4. _____
5. _____
6. _____
7. _____

18/46
* stay out of the sun
  between 10:00 a.m.
  and 2:00 p.m.
* limit your use of
  sun lamps and tanning
  salons
* always use sunscreen
  with PABA to block
  ultraviolet rays
* examine your entire
  body once a year for
  suspicious moles
Prevention
Page #461

Identify three things you can do to
protect yourself from skin cancer.
1. _____
2. _____
3. _____

18/47   * you have a family   Name three indicators of the need for
           history of diabetes   a yearly blood glucose test.
         * you are over age 40   1. _____
         * you are clearly over-   2. _____
           weight   3. _____
         * you have given birth
           to a baby that weighs
           more than 9 pounds
         Major Illnesses
         Page #468

18/48   * stay alert, don't get   Identify four rules for safe driving.
           too comfortable   1. _____
         * keep racing fantasies   2. _____
           to yourself   3. _____
         * use rearview mirror   4. _____
           often
         * keep a safe distance
           between you and the
           car in front
         * whenever possible,
           leave yourself a way
           out of the immediate
           driving situation
         Accidents
         Page #474

18/49   * don't smoke   Name four strategies for reducing the
         * eat right (low fat)   risk of serious disease and accidents.
         * exercise regularly   1. _____
         * have regular screen-   2. _____
           ing tests   3. _____
         * proceed with caution   4. _____
           on land and water
         Prevention
         Page #478

Chapter 18: Cancer, Major Illnesses, and Accidents

Matching

18/50   Directions: Match each of the cancer terms on the left with its correct definition on the right. Each definition may be used only once.

	Term		Definition
1.	__ remission	a.	cancerous
2.	__ neoplasm	b.	invasion or replacement of healthy cells
3.	__ benign	c.	asymptomatic state when spread of cancerous cells appears stopped
4.	__ malignant	d.	a substance that promotes cancerous growth
5.	__ infiltration	e.	new growth, or tumor
6.	__ metastasize	f.	spread to other parts of the body
		g.	slightly abnormal or non-threatening cells

1-c, 2-e, 3-g,
4-a, 5-b, 6-f
Cancer
Pages #451-452

18/51   Directions: Match each of the screening tests on the left with its correct schedule on the right. Each schedule may be used only once.

	Test		Schedule
1.	__ mammogram	a.	every six months
2.	__ pap test (pap smear)	b.	every year after age 50
3.	__ digital rectal exam	c.	one baseline between ages 35 and 39; every 1-2 years from ages 40-49; yearly after age 50
4.	__ proctosigmoidoscopy	d.	yearly after age 40
5.	__ stool blood test	e.	every 3-5 years after age 50
		f.	every year after becoming sexually active

1-c, 2-f, 3-d,
4-e, 5-b
Prevention
Pages #455-456

<u>Essay</u>

18/52   Why do you think cancer is called a "lifestyle" disease?

18/53   Despite the advances made in the treatment and prevention of cancer,
         there always seem to be a number of experimental or highly
         controversial treatments not generally available. Oftentimes, those
         stricken with cancer will try anything, including traveling to
         another country to obtain drugs or treatment unavailable in the U.S.
         Do you think seriously ill or terminal cancer patients should have
         access to experimental or controversial treatments? If yes, under
         what conditions? If not, why not?

18/54   Which of the major health issues in this chapter do you believe
         constitutes the greatest problem for the U.S. health care system?
         Defend your answer.

18/55   Many experts acknowledge that a "safe" automobile <u>could</u> be built;
         one that provides a high degree of protection from injury during an
         accident, and whose design reflects passenger safety concerns more
         than marketing appeal or horsepower. Why do you think such a car
         has never been built? Does the automobile industry share any of the
         responsiblility for the high number of serious injuries and
         fatalities suffered on our highways each year? If so, what
         responsibility do they have? If not, why not?

AN INVITATION TO HEALTH
TEST BANK

Section V - Understanding Your Risks

Chapter 19: Immunity and Infectious Diseases

In this chapter -

*   Infectious Diseases
*   Immune Disorders
*   AIDS
*   Sexually Transmitted Diseases

Section V - Understanding Your Risks
Chapter 19: Immunity and Infectious Diseases -
Protecting Yourself

True-False

19/1	True Infectious Diseases Page #481	The infections most threatening to the public's health today are sexually transmitted diseases.
19/2	True Immune System Page #481	The body's immune response is triggered by the presence of pathogens.
19/3	False Immune System Page #482	In addition to providing extra energy during a crisis, adrenalin boosts the body's immune response.
19/4	True Infection Process Page #483	The biological or physical means of transmission by which a pathogen is brought into contact with the host is called a vector.
19/5	False Infection Process Page #484	Antibiotics are an effective treatment against viruses.
19/6	True Infection Process Page #483	Viruses are unable to reproduce by themselves.
19/7	True Infection Process Page #484	Most kinds of bacteria do not cause disease.
19/8	False Infectious Diseases Page #484	There is a single virus that causes colds and flu.
19/9	True Infectious Diseases Page #489	Children and teenagers who take aspirin for colds or flu risk contracting a potentially fatal condition known as Reye's syndrome.
19/10	False Infectious Diseases Page #491	There is no safe, effective vaccine against hepatitis B.
19/11	False Infectious Diseases Page #492	The availability of vaccines has virtually eliminated deaths due to vaccine-preventable diseases.

19/12	True Immune Disorders Page #493	An allergy, or hypersensitivity to a substance in the environment, is a form of immune disorder.
19/13	True AIDS Page #494	Most deaths related to acquired immune deficiency syndrome (AIDS) are not caused by the AIDS virus itself, but by certain infections or cancers against which the body can no longer defend itself.
19/14	False AIDS Page #495	Acquired immune deficiency syndrome (AIDS) can be caught through casual contact with an infected person.
19/15	True AIDS Page #496	Women and children of black and Hispanic origin have a disproportionately high incidence of AIDS infection.
19/16	True AIDS Page #498	There is currently no effective treatment for AIDS.
19/17	True Sexually Transmitted Diseases Page #500	The incidence of sexually transmitted diseases among teenagers aged 15 to 19 years outnumbers the total for all other groups combined.
19/18	True Sexually Transmitted Diseases Page #506	Both gonorrhea and syphilis can develop into serious, life-threatening infections if left untreated.
19/19	True Sexually Transmitted Diseases Page #507	Syphilis can be caught by kissing an infected person.
19/20	False Sexually Transmitted Diseases Page #507	Herpes Simplex Type 2 is the most commonly transmitted bacteria among heterosexual white Americans.

<u>Mulitple Choice</u>

19/21   b
         Immune Response
         Pages #482-483

The body's immune response can be characterized by all of the following except

a. lymphocytes and macrophages are stored in lymph nodes.
b. each person's immune response is the same.
c. the spread of pathogens into the blood causes systemic disease.
d. the basic machinery for fighting infection is a variety of different immune cells.

19/22   a
         Immune Response
         Page #482

Active immunity

a. is acquired when the body makes its own antibodies to a pathogen.
b. is produced using injections of gamma globulin from an immune source.
c. is usually temporary.
d. is always more effective than passive immunity.

19/23   d
         Infection Process
         Pages #483-484

Which of the following is <u>not</u> capable of causing an infection?

a. bacteria
b. protozoa
c. virus
d. T-cell

19/24   d
         Infection Process
         Page #483

A virus attacks the body

a. by releasing poisonous enzymes that destroy cells.
b. by multiplying outside of cells in the blood, then attacking certain organs.
c. by competing with the host for nutrients.
d. by using the reproductive elements of existing cells to manufacture new virus.

19/25   d   Major methods of infection transmission
            Infection Process   include food, water, person to person
            Page #485   contact, and

                                     a. air.
                                     b. blood transfusions.
                                     c. mother to fetus transmission.
                                     d. animal vectors.

19/26   a   Mild, generalized symptoms such as
            Infection Process   headache and irritability are common
            Page #486   during the period of infection called

                                     a. prodromal.
                                     b. incubation.
                                     c. recovery.
                                     d. illness.

19/27   c   Which of the following statements about
            Infectious Diseases   influenza is most accurate?
            Page #489
                                     a. There is currently a safe, effective
                                        treatment for the flu virus.
                                     b. Aspirin is the medication of choice
                                        for children and teenagers with flu
                                        symptoms.
                                     c. Flu viruses are especially conta-
                                        gious during the first 3 days of the
                                        disease.
                                     d. The side effects of flu vaccines are
                                        not a significant factor in deter-
                                        mining who should be vaccinated.

19/28   b   With regard to the major infectious
            Infectious Diseases   diseases, which of the following state-
            Page #490   ments is most accurate?

                                     a. 80 million Americans have the tuber-
                                        culosis bacillus in their body.
                                     b. The primary symptom of Chronic
                                        Epstein-Barr virus is exhaustion.
                                     c. Mononucleosis can not be caught by
                                        kissing.
                                     d. Hepatitis B is rarely transmitted
                                        through sexual contact.

19/29   b
        Infectious Diseases
        Page #491

Toxic shock syndrome (TSS) is a potentially fatal disease

a. that is always associated with the
   use of high absorbency tampons.
b. in which the body's blood pressure
   falls to a level that cannot sustain
   life.
c. that recurrs in about 50% of its
   victims.
d. whose high rate of recurrence cannot
   be prevented by switching to external forms of menstrual protection.

19/30   d
        Infectious Diseases
        Page #492

The four diseases for which immuniza-
tion is most essential are polio,
tetanus, measles, and

a. hepatitis.
b. mononucleosis.
c. tuberculosis.
d. diphtheria.

19/31   c
        Immune Disorders
        Page #494

Myasthenia gravis, rheumatoid arthritis, and lupus erythematosus are all
examples of

a. allergies.
b. immune deficiencies.
c. autoimmune disorders.
d. viral infections.

19/32   a
        AIDS
        Page #495

Which of the following statements about
the spread of AIDS is not accurate?

a. The rate of new infections among
   homosexuals is rising rapidly, according to the Centers for Disease
   Control.
b. The Public Health Service estimates
   between 1.5 and 2 million Americans
   are infected with the AIDS virus.
c. The Centers for Disease Control
   estimates that 179,000 people will
   have died from AIDS by 1995.
d. The World Health Organization estimates that 10 million people world-
   wide may be infected with the AIDS
   virus.

19/33   c
           AIDS
           Page #496

The behavior most likely to transmit the AIDS virus is

a. working closely with an AIDS carrier.
b. oral sex with an infected partner.
c. sharing a needle used by an infected person.
d. donating blood in a major, metropolitan area.

19/34   a
           AIDS
           Page #494

Most epidemiologists believe that the AIDS virus first infected humans in

a. Africa.
b. Haiti.
c. New York City.
d. Canada.

19/35   c
           AIDS
           Page #496

With regard to groups at risk for AIDS,

a. IV drug users represent the largest group of infected persons in the United States.
b. in Africa, AIDS is spread primarily through homosexual contact.
c. the risk of infection following exposure depends, in part, on heredity and previous infections with diseases like hepatitis.
d. most children with AIDS are white.

19/36   b
           AIDS
           Page #497

Health officials recommend AIDS testing for members of all the following groups except

a. women who have had sex with bisexual men.
b. anyone who has received a blood transfusion from 1985-1988.
c. anyone who has had sex with an IV drug user.
d. men who have had multiple, anonymous sex partners and are worried about being infected.

19/37   d
           AIDS
           Page #498

The drug AZT

a. has few significant side effects.
b. is relatively inexpensive to obtain.
c. is effective for less than half of those taking it.
d. temporarily improves the quality of life for certain people with AIDS.

19/38   c
           STD's
           Page #500

Each of the following are true of sexually transmitted diseases except

a. STD pathogens flourish in warm,
   dark, and moist body surfaces.
b. curing one STD does not mean you
   have cured all other STD's with
   which you may be infected.
c. it is not possible to have more than
   one STD at a time.
d. STD's are the major cause of preventable sterility in America.

19/39   b
           STD's
           Page #500

Which of the following statements about
gonorrhea is least accurate?

a. Infection is generally more notice-
   able in men than women.
b. Sexual intercourse is the only means
   of transmission.
c. Gonorrhea is the leading cause of
   sterility in women.
d. Some strains of gonorrhea are resis-
   tant to penicillin.

19/40   a
           STD's
           Page #506

The stage at which a lesion, or chancre
appears during a syphilis infections is

a. the primary stage.
b. the secondary stage.
c. the latent stage.
d. the late stage.

19/41   c
           STD's
           Page #507

Which of the following groups are <u>not</u>
at high risk for chlamydia?

a. aged 24 years or younger
b. users of birth control pills or
   other nonbarrier methods
c. homosexuals and lesbians
d. engaging in sex with one or more
   new partners within the preceeding
   2 months

19/42   b
           STD's
           Pages #508

Chlamydia and nongonococcal urethritis
(NGU)

a. are both consequences of gonorrhea.
b. are both generally asymptomatic in
   women (do <u>not</u> present symptoms).
c. can both be treated effectively with
   penicillin.
d. are transmitted exclusively through
   sexual intercourse.

Chapter 19: **Immunity and Infectious Diseases**

19/43   d
         STD's
         Page #508

Herpes simplex

a. affects less than 5% of the sexually active population.
b. can be cured with antibiotics.
c. does not pose a risk to the fetus of an infected woman.
d. can be controlled, but not cured, with the prescription drug Acyclovir (ACV).

19/44   c
         Urinary/Reproductive
         Infections
         Page #511

Trichomoniasis, cystitis, and acute pyelonephritis are all

a. types of sexually transmitted disease.
b. consequences of sexually transmitted diseases.
c. infections of the reproductive or urinary systems.
d. opportunistic infections that affect people with AIDS.

Completion

19/45   * get enough vitamins and minerals in your diet
         * avoid fatty foods
         * get enough sleep
         * exercise regularly
         * get moderate exposure to the sun, use sunscreen
         * don't smoke
         * if you drink alcohol, do so in moderation
         * don't use drugs
         Immune System
         Page #482

What are four things you can do to bolster your immunity?
1. _____
2. _____
3. _____
4. _____

19/46   * drink lots of liquids, but not alcohol
         * stay inside as long as you have a fever
         * take aspirin for pain unless you're a teenager
         * rest as much as possible
         * avoid exposure to other illnesses
         Infectious Diseases
         Page #490

What are four ways to speed up your recovery from mononucleosis?
1. _____
2. _____
3. _____
4. _____

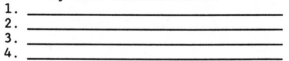

228

19/47   * fevers or night sweats
      * swollen lymph nodes in
        neck, groin, underarm
      * weakness, fatigue
      * diarrhea
      * white spots in mouth
      * herpes sore that won't
        go away
      * purple or dark red lumps
        on body that keep growing
      * headaches, dry cough
      * confusion, coordination
        problems
      * infections of skin and
        chest
      AIDS
      Page #497

Identify six symptoms of AIDS.
1. _____
2. _____
3. _____
4. _____
5. _____
6. _____

19/48   * <u>always</u> use safer-sex
        practices such as con-
        doms and spermicides
        with nonoxynol-9
      * donate your own blood
        prior to surgery
      * avoid casual, multiple
        sexual contacts
      * don't share implements
        that might be contamin-
        ated with blood from an
        infected person
      * use caution in any situa-
        tion that involves the
        piercing of skin or
        mucous membranes
      * use proper safety pre-
        cautions at work if you
        are at risk for exposure
        to the AIDS virus
      AIDS
      Page #499

What are four things you can do to
protect yourself from AIDS?
1. _____
2. _____
3. _____
4. _____

Matching

19/49   Directions: Match each component of the body's immune system on the
         left with its correct description on the right. Each description may
         be used only once.

         Immune System Component   Description
1. __ Complement   a. large scavenger cells that "eat"
2. __ Interferons   diseased or run-down red blood cells
3. __ Lymphocytes (white   b. lymphocytes that mature in the bone
       blood cells)   marrow and produce antibodies
4. __ B-cells   c. enzymes that burn through bacterial
5. __ T-cells   cell membranes
6. __ Macrophages   d. the smallest type of antigen
7. __ Natural Killer (NK)   e. protein substance that inactivates
       cells   invading viruses
                                          f. lymphocytes that attack tumors and
                                             virus-infected cells
                                          g. lymphocytes that mature in the
                                             thymus and activate other immune
                                             cells
                                          h. cells that patrol the bloodstream
                                             destroying foreign bodies

         1-c, 2-e, 3-h, 4-b
         5-g, 6-a, 7-f
         Immune System
         Page #482

19/50   Directions: Match each of the virus types on the left with its correct
         description on the right. Each description may be used only once.

              Virus Type   Description
1   __ Rhinovirus/Adenovirus   a. causes several forms of liver infec-
2.   __ Influenza   tion
3.   __ Herpesvirus   b. give no early indication of their
4.   __ Papillomavirus   presence, but cause rare, fatal dis-
5.   __ Hepatitis   eases within a few years
6.   __ Slow Virus   c. cause upper-respiratory-tract
7.   __ Retrovirus   infections
                                    d. competes with body for nutrients
                                    e. replicates backward compared to
                                       other viruses; unusual in humans
                                       except for AIDS patients
                                    f. causes few symptoms, but has been
                                       linked to cervical cancer
                                    g. causes genital sores and fever
                                       blisters
                                    h. able to change protein coats and
                                       prevent development of resistance

         1-c, 2-h, 3-g, 4-f,
         5-a, 6-b, 7-e,
         Infection Process
         Pages #483-484

Chapter 19: Immunity and Infectious
Diseases

19/51   Directions: Match each of the sexually transmitted diseases (STD's) on the left with its correct set of symptoms on the right. Each set of symptoms may be used only once.

<u>STD</u>
1. __ Gonorrhea
2. __ Syphilis
3. __ Chlamydia
4. __ Nongonococcal Urethritis
5. __ Herpes Simplex
6. __ Chancroid
7. __ Granuloma Inguinale
8. __ Lymphogranuloma Venerum

<u>Symptoms</u>
a. chancre or lesion during primary stage; rash, fever, sores, and ultimately blindness or insanity
b. painful urination; thick, yellow-white pus oozing from penis in men, most women may have no symptoms at all
c. genital lesions/blisters, strong psychological impact (depression)
d. small lesion near site of infection, followed by swollen or ruptured lymph nodes, fever, and joint pain
e. symptoms similar to gonorrhea; may include itching or vaginal discharge in women
f. painful urination and clear, watery discharge from penis; most women experience no symptoms, some develop vaginal discharge or bleeding and painful urination
g. painless warts that appear on or near genitals
h. soft, very painful ulcers that bleed easily and ooze pus; may spread to lymph glands and produce swelling
i. small, rounded, pus-filled ulcerations on skin of external genitals; can spread and become chronic

1-b, 2-a, 3-f, 4-e,
5-c, 6-h, 7-i, 8-d
STD's
Pages #504-505

Essay

19/52   Success in preventing sexually transmitted diseases depends to a large extent on behavior changes by members of groups at risk. Frequently, the messages our society sends to sexually active people are confusing and contradictory. On one hand, being sexually attractive is highly valued and sought after. On the other hand, exercising sexual freedom carries with it a number of serious health risks (both physical and emotional). Although many people argue that this kind of information and socialization ought to take place in the home, a large number of sexually active young adults remains poorly informed about the health risks of sexual activity. If it were up to you, how would you ensure that sexually active young people were thoroughly educated and capable of responsible sexual relationships?

19/53   Funding for AIDS research and treatment has grown slowly since its discovery in 1981, and remains inadequate according to many health experts. Yet, health care officials must make decisions about where these limited resources should be used. If you had to apportion the available AIDS funding between 1) research to develop a vaccine to prevent AIDS and 2) research to develop a cure, how would you allocate the money? What are the criteria for your decision?

19/54   Consider the following statement:

"During the 20th century, the single greatest contribution to the enhancement of the quality of life in the United States has been the virtual elimination of serious infectious diseases such as smallpox, diphtheria, tuberculosis, etc."

Take a position for or against this statement, and defend your point of view.

19/55   A friend has confided in you that their AIDS blood test came back positive, and they aren't sure what to do next. What advice would you give them?

AN INVITATION TO HEALTH
TEST BANK

Section V - Understanding Your Risks

Chapter 20: The Environment's Impact

In this chapter -

*   Environmental Hazards
*   Air Pollution
*   Indoor Pollution
*   Water Pollution
*   Chemical Pollution
*   Noise Pollution
*   Impact of Pollution
*   Violence
*   Nuclear Waste

Section V - Understanding Your Risks
Chapter 20: The Environment's Impact

True-False

20/1	True Environmental Hazards Page #515	In order for a change in the air, soil, or water to be classified as pollution, the change must reduce the ability to support life.
20/2	True Environmental Hazards Page #515	For most people, the worksite is the most likely place to encounter an environmental hazard.
20/3	False Air Pollution Page #516	Most sources of air pollution are natural, such as smoke and dust.
20/4	True Air Pollution Page #516	Gray air, or sulfur dioxide smog, is common to the eastern United States and Europe.
20/5	True Air Pollution Page #517	The direct consequence of the depletion of the earth's ozone layer is an increase in the strength of ultraviolet radiation at ground level.
20/6	True Indoor Pollution Page #518	Indoor pollution is largely a result of the materials used in building and furnishing a home.
20/7	True Water Pollution Page #520	Drinking chlorinated water (water treated with chlorine to kill bacteria) has been associated with increased risk for certain types of cancer.
20/8	True Chemical Pollution Page #520	Little is known about the health risks of most common chemicals in use today.
20/9	False Chemical Pollution Page #520	Pesticides containing chlorinated hydrocarbons such as DDT break down rapidly in the environment.
20/10	True Chemical Pollution Page #521	Mercury metal is poisonous only if it is vaporized and inhaled.
20/11	True Chemical Pollution Page #521	The primary cause of lead in the atmosphere is the combustion of leaded gasoline.

20/12	False Chemical Pollution Pages #523-524	Burial of toxic waste is a safe and effective method of long-term waste disposal.
20/13	True Noise Pollution Page #524	The primary cause of hearing disorders is exposure to excess noise.
20/14	True Impact of Pollution Page #526	Americans make up about 6% of the world's population and use a third of the world's mineral and energy resources.
20/15	False Impact of Pollution Pages #526-527	The majority of countries in the world are capable of growing or buying enough food to feed their populations.
20/16	True Violence Page #528	Violence is the leading cause of death among adolescents in the United States.
20/17	True Violence Page #529	Murders within the family account for 30% of the total number of murders annually.
20/18	False Nuclear Risks Page #529	A significant portion of the radiation in our environment is produced by commercial power plants.
20/19	True Nuclear Risks Page #531	30-50% of all X-rays taken by doctors each year are unnecessary, according to the Environmental Protecion Agency.
20/20	True Nuclear Risks Page #533	After 30 years of service, nuclear reactors must be dismantled because they are no longer safe to operate.

Multiple Choice

20/21	a Environmental Hazards Page #518	Exposure to asbestos over many years may cause lung disease. Asbestos poisoning is the consequence of a. anthropogenic pollution. b. acute exposure. c. exposure to teratogens. d. natural pollution.

20/22   c
Environmental Hazards
Page #515

The effects of pollution depend on each of the following except

a. the duration of exposure.
b. the chemical nature of the pollut-ant.
c. whether the pollutant is natural or manmade.
d. the concentration of the pollutant.

20/23   d
Air Pollution
Page #516

Which of the following statements about air pollution is most accurate?

a. Sulfur-dioxide pollution has increased during the past 10 years.
b. Ozone is a byproduct of gray-air smog.
c. Carbon-monoxide levels increased during the period 1965-1985.
d. Particulate pollution has decreased during the past 10 years.

20/24   b
Air Pollution
Page #517

Chlorofluorocarbons

a. pose significant health risks for people who spend a great deal of time indoors near refrigerators and air conditioning units.
b. continue to be released into the atmosphere in amounts that are depleting the ozone layer.
c. production was banned totally by all 24 nations participating in the 1987 Montreal conference.
d. cause skin cancer directly when they come into contact with the skin.

20/25   a
Indoor Pollution
Page #519

Indoor pollution risks

a. have been difficult to determine because of uncertainty regarding the extent and harmful effects of the pollution.
b. drop dramatically if you live in a new, tightly sealed house.
c. are generally the same, regardless of the geographical location of the building.
d. have resulted in the removal of asbestos from all public schools.

20/26   d
         Chemical Pollution
         Pages #519-523

Which of the following is <u>not</u> a type of chemical pesticide?

a. carbamates
b. organic phosphates
c. chlorinated hydrocarbons
d. chlorofluorocarbons

20/27   c
         Chemical Pollution
         Page #521

Lead

a. is toxic only at high levels of exposure.
b. in the atmosphere is primarily the product of industrial and commercial pollution.
c. levels in the atmosphere have risen only in or near sites of industrial development.
d. oxide is still an ingredient in many paint pigments.

20/28   b
         Chemical Pollution
         Page #522

Long-term exposure to dioxin may result in all of the following except

a. birth defects.
b. mental retardation.
c. damage to the immune system.
d. tumors.

20/29   c
         Noise Pollution
         Page #525

The upper limit of hearing safety is about

a. 30-40 decibels.
b. 40-50 decibels.
c. 80-90 decibels.
d. anything over 100 decibels.

20/30   a
         Impact of Population
         Page #526

The primary factor affecting the pollution of our environment is

a. our planet's population.
b. the lopsided consumption of energy resources by industrialized nations.
c. the emergence of larger and larger cities.
d. the use of non-biodegradable packaging.

20/31   d
Violence
Page #520

All of the following are factors that contribute to the likelihood of wife abuse except

a. the husband's use of alcohol.
b. whether or not the husband was raised in an abusive home.
c. the husband's level of stress and frustration.
d. the husband's level of self-control.

20/32   a
Violence
Page #528

Child abuse

a. incidents are on the rise.
b. incidents are decreasing in number.
c. is not related to the psychological state of the abuser.
d. is unrelated to the abuser's experiences as a child.

20/33   c
Nuclear Risks
Page #529

In the measurement of radiation,

a. a rad is a measure of the biological effect of radiation exposure.
b. the amount of biological damage is unrelated to the type of radiation.
c. a rem is the measure of the biological effect of radiation exposure.
d. the effect of low-level exposure has been precisely determined.

20/34   c
Nuclear Risks
Page #531

The most hazardous type of radioactivity is

a. Alpha particles.
b. microwaves.
c. Gamma rays.
d. Beta particles

20/35   d
Nuclear Risks
Page #532

Effective and safe disposal of radioactive wastes

a. can be accomplished by storing them in the cooling water bath at nuclear reactor sites.
b. is made easier by the fact that most waste products stop emitting radiation after about 20 years.
c. has posed a potential health problem for only the last 10-15 years.
d. is complicated by the fact that there now exist more than 3 billion cubic feet of radioactive waste.

Completion

20/36   * don't buy a home insu-
lated with formaldehyde
* if your home is insulat-
ed with formaldehyde,
keep heat and humidity
down; use air condition-
ers and dehumidifiers
* keep your house well-
ventilated
* seal wood products with
formaldehyde sealant
* have your house checked
by your local health
department
Indoor Pollution
Page #518

What are three things you can do to
protect yourself from formaldehyde?
1. _____
2. _____
3. _____

20/37   * inspect your house be-
before renovating
* don't touch any loose
asbestos
* don't rely on air tests
to determine if asbes-
tos is present
* if you find asbestos in
your house, consider
sealing it rather than
removing it
Indoor Pollution
Page #518

What are two things you can do to
protect yourself from asbestos?
1. _____
2. _____

20/38   * limit your use of aero-
sols
* vent all gas ovens to
the outside
* seal all materials con-
taining formaldehyde or
radon
* air your house out as
often as possible,
especially in winter
* consider buying a heat
exchanger as a method
for heating/cooling
your home
Indoor Pollution
Page #520

Identify three ways to reduce indoor
pollution.
1. _____
2. _____
3. _____

20/39
* read the label care-
fully
* store products in a
locked place
* don't measure pesti-
cides with food prep-
aration utensils
* don't mix chemicals
with each other
* wear rubber gloves
* store only in the manu-
facturer's container
* hire licensed extermi-
nators only; check
their work carefully;
don't let them use
chlordane; stay away
from the house during
the fumigation
Chemical Pollution
Page #521

Name four tips for using pesticides
safely.
1. _____
2. _____
3. _____

20/40
* find out about any toxic
spills that have
occurred near her home
* limit her intake of
freshwater sportfish
such as carp, salmon,
lake trout, & perch
* don't crash diet while
breast-feeding
* if she thinks she has
been exposed, get a
blood test as soon as
possible and discuss
the results with her
doctor
Chemical Pollution
Page #523

Your friend, who is pregnant and
wants to nurse her baby, has expressed
concern about protecting her baby
from chemical pollutants. What are
three things she can do?
1. _____
2. _____
3. _____

20/41
* make sure you have the
right address
* identify the bill or
issue you are addres-
sing
* write before the bill
comes up for a vote
* concentrate on your
representative
* be as brief and to the
point as possible
* use your own words
* give reasons for your
position
* don't threaten
Chemical Pollution
Page #524

Writing your government representatives
is an effective way to fight for a
clean, safe environment. Identify five
ways to make your letter more effective.
1. _____
2. _____
3. _____
4. _____
5. _____

20/42   * wear hearing protectors to prevent exposure to dangerous levels of noise
* limit your exposure to loud noise
* be careful when wearing Walkman-type stereos
* have your hearing checked regularly
* keep your home quiet

Noise Pollution
Page #525

What are three ways you can protect your ears from noise pollution?
1. _____
2. _____
3. _____

20/43   * ask why the X-ray is being ordered
* keep a good record of all X-ray exams
* ask the radiologist to explain how much radiation you will be exposed to
* don't refuse a needed X-ray just because you are worried about the effects

Nuclear Risks
Page #531

Identify two ways you can avoid unnecessary X-rays.
1. _____
2. _____
3. _____

20/44   * recycle paper and glass
* drive a fuel-efficient automobile
* don't litter
* keep your radio/stereo at a reasonably low volume
* buy products with bio-degradable packaging
* turn out the ligts when leaving a room
* don't let faucets drip or leak
* don't use aerosol sprays
* buy energy-efficient appliances
* be an active consumer

Healthy Environment
Page #534

Name seven ways to protect your environment.
1. _____
2. _____
3. _____
4. _____
5. _____
6. _____
7. _____

Matching

20/45   Directions: Match each of the environmental terms on the left with
its correct definition on the right. Each definition may be used
only once.

                Term

1. __ anthropogenic
2. __ acute effect
3. __ chronic effect
4. __ pollution
5. __ mutagen
6. __ teratogen

Definition

a. agents that cross the placenta
and cause spontaneous abortion or
birth defects
b. a severe, immediate reaction,
usually after a single large exposure
c. changes that reduce the ability to
support life
d. a combination of smoke and fog
e. agents that trigger changes in
genetic material
f. a recurrent or constant reaction
following repeated exposures
g. caused by human activities

1-g, 2-b, 3-f,
4-c, 5-e, 6-a
Environmental Hazards
Page #515

Essay

20/46   Most types of industry generate waste products. While safe and
effective methods of disposal may differ, they are frequently
expensive and time-consuming if performed properly. Should the
producers of waste products be <u>totally</u> responsible for their safe
and effective disposal (as opposed to temporary storage or dumping)?
If so, should the cost of disposing of these waste be passed along
to the consumer in the form of price increases? Why, or why not?

20/47   Rapid population growth is clearly a problem in a number of
developing nations. China has had some measure of success in
managing the rate of growth of its population; other countries have
been less effective. What do you see as the obstacles to managing
population growth effectively and fairly? What should be done to
overcome these obstacles?

20/48   Very little, if anything, is known about the health effects of the
majority of chemicals commonly in use today in the U.S. Do you
think federal and state governments are doing enough to protect
consumers from the potentially harmful effects associated with the
use of these substances?   If it were up to you, how would you
ensure that products in the marketplace were safe to use?

20/49   Sooner or later, Americans are going to have to give up their
         gasoline-powered automobile engines in exchange for electrical
         motors or other alternatives. Some experts believe that a
         pollution-free automobile engine could be built today if the
         political and economic "climate" was more pro-environment. Do you
         think the automobile industry is doing all it can to
         reduce/eliminate automobile pollution? Why have we continued to
         build and use a type of engine that is so harmful to our
         environment?

20/50   What is the most significant pollution problem our country faces
         today? Why? What could you as an individual do to improve the
         situation?

Section V - Understanding Your Risks

<u>Chapter 21: Coming to Terms with Death</u>

In this chapter -

* Death
* Dying
* Grief
* Practicalities
* Preparation

Section V - Understanding Your Risks
Chapter 21: Coming to Terms with Death

True-False

21/1	True Death Page #537	Brain death, or the irreversible cessation of all functioning of the brain, is the criteria used by most states in determining legally if death has occurred.
21/2	True Denial Page #537	Some denial of death is necessary in order for us to concentrate on daily living activities.
21/3	False Dying Page #537	Most people with a terminal illness would rather not know the truth about their condition.
21/4	True Dying Page #538	Elisabeth Kubler-Ross has identified five stages of emotional reaction to impending death.
21/5	False Dying Page #539	According to Edwin Schneidman, the way in which we deal with our own impending death is unrelated to the way in which we have handled previous crises.
21/6	True Dying Page #539	Dying patients over 50 years of age are less distressed mentally and physically than those under age 50.
21/7	False Grief Page #541	Grief has few, if any, significant physiological effects.
21/8	True Grief Page #543	Grieving is necessary in order to return to a normal psychological state of love and hope.
21/9	False Grief Page #544	The majority of bereaved people need professional, psychological counseling.
21/10	True Practicalities Page #545	For some survivors, a funeral helps them mourn their loss and come to terms with what has happened.

21/11   True
         Practicalities
         Page #545

The primary difference between a funeral and a memorial service is that the body of the deceased is not present at a memorial service.

21/12   False
         Practicalities
         Page #545

Medical/educational autopsies may be performed without the consent of the deceased person's family.

21/13   False
         Preparation
         Page #546

"Living Wills" are legally binding in all 50 states.

21/14   True
         Preparation
         Page #548

If you die without a will, the state you live in will decide what to do with your property and/or children.

21/15   True
         Preparation
         Page #549

You must be 18 years of age or older in order for your organ donor card to be valid.

Multiple Choice

21/16   c
         Death
         Page #537

The traditional legal definition of death (failure of heart or lungs to function) is inadequate because

a. the cells in these organs may be alive even when they are no longer functioning.
b. it doesn't take into account the spirit's departure from the body.
c. these functions may be maintained artificially, even if the brain is "dead."
d. these organs can usually be revived.

21/17   b
         Denial
         Page #537

All of the following are true regarding the denial of death except

a. most people engage in denial to some degree.
b. the immediacy of the threat of death is unrelated to the degree of denial.
c. it exists even in the face of clear proof that death is likely.
d. some degree of denial can enhance one's experience of life.

21/18   d
        Dying
        Page #538

With regard to the emotional stages of grief described by Elisabeth Kubler-Ross,

a. each stage appears independently of the others.
b. each stage takes about the same amount of time, usually several days.
c. the stages always occur in the same sequence.
d. denial may recur at any time.

21/19   a
        Dying
        Page #539

Which of the following statements regarding Edwin Schneidman's work on death is least accurate?

a. He agrees with Kubler-Ross that denial of death occurs as a single, well-defined stage.
b. He believes that the five-stage theory of Kubler-Ross is too simplistic.
c. He believes that people respond to imminent death in a way similar to previous major stressful events.
d. He believes that denial comes and goes during the period before death.

21/20   c
        Dying
        Page #539

People who are dying

a. do not usually share common physical symptoms.
b. in a hospital are just as alert and free of physical distress as those who are dying at home.
c. and have weak religious convictions show more fear than those with strong, or total absence of, religious beliefs.
d. are usually more afraid of death itself than the suffering associated with dying.

21/21   a
        Dying
        Page #539

Researchers are studying new ways to relieve pain using all of the following restricted drugs except

a. cocaine.
b. heroin.
c. LSD.
d. marijuana.

21/22   d
         Dying
         Page #540

Hopsice patients

a. are similar to other dying patients
   except they receive treatments to
   cure their disease at home.
b. usually have a life expectancy of
   1-3 years.
c. cannot be reimbursed for hospice
   services by insurance companies.
d. are considered terminal, and
   treated to make their life pain-free
   and comfortable.

21/23   b
         Dying
         Page #540

Which of the following statements about
dying is most accurate?

a. Dying patients cannot legally refuse
   life-sustaining treatment.
b. Euthanasia, or "mercy death," is
   illegal.
c. Euthanasia is the witholding of
   life-sustaining treatment such as
   oxygen or intravenous feeding.
d. Dyathanasia usually occurs when a
   physician administers a large dose
   of pain relieving medicine that
   causes the patient's heart and
   breathing to stop.

21/24   c
         Dying
         Page #541

Suicide

a. is rarely seen in terminally ill
   patients.
b. is not among the top ten causes
   of death in the U.S.
c. attempts outnumber completed suicides by as much as 40 to 1.
d. is unrelated to depression.

21/25   d
         Grief
         Page #541

All of the following are true regarding
the death of an immediate family member
except

a. a recent survey of college students
   showed death of a family member as
   being their greatest fear.
b. it produces a wide range of feelings
   and reactions among family members.
c. about 8 million Americans experience
   the death of a family member each
   year.
d. the family's feelings are not affected by age of the deceased person.

21/26   b   The impact of death on survivors
         Grief
         Page #542   a. includes major disruptions of one's
                                       life for only about 3 months.
                                    b. is greatest for those with poor
                                       mental health and a lack of social
                                       support.
                                    c. is generally more severe for women
                                       over age 75 than for men.
                                    d. is not affected by the suddenness of
                                       the death.

21/27   a   Which of the following statements about
         Grief   a child's experience of death is most
         Page #542   accurate?

                                    a. Loss of a parent frequently results
                                       in major psychiatric disorders later
                                       in life.
                                    b. By the age of three, most children
                                       understand that death is the end of
                                       life and is inevitable.
                                    c. Children express their feelings
                                       about death directly and clearly.
                                    d. Children do not experience grief
                                       for people outside of the immediate
                                       family.

21/28   c   The primary difference between "normal"
         Grief   grief and "pathologic" grief is that
         Page #543
                                    a. normal grief is always resolved
                                       within 1-2 years.
                                    b. pathologic grief is usually associ-
                                       ated with the absence of feelings.
                                    c. pathologic grief victims get "stuck"
                                       in the process of resolving their
                                       feelings.
                                    d. normal grief involves clinging,
                                       denial, avoidance, and excess at-
                                       tachment.

21/29   d   Memorial societies provide all of the
         Practicalities   following services except
         Page #544
                                    a. planning in advance for death.
                                    b. obtaining services at moderate
                                       cost.
                                    c. easing the emotional burden of the
                                       family and friends.
                                    d. advocating elaborate arrangements
                                       in honor of the deceased.

21/30   a
          Preparation
          Page #546

Which of the following is the <u>least</u> important reason to write a holographic will?

a. You expect to inherit some money when a rich relative dies.
b. You have children.
c. You are married.
d. You own property.

Completion

21/31   * denial
          * anger
          * bargaining
          * depression
          * acceptance
          Dying
          Page #538

What are the five stages of emotional reaction to impending death identified by Elisabeth Kubler-Ross?
1. _____
2. _____
3. _____
4. _____
5. _____

21/32   * visit with the person;
            don't leave them alone
          * don't worry about
            saying the right thing
          * listen
          * be genuine
          * don't try to explain
            or rationalize what
            has happened
          Dying
          Page #539

What are three things you can do to comfort a dying person?
1. _____
2. _____
3. _____

21/33   * don't try to hide your
            own sadness
          * don't convey a sense of
            anxiety about the
            future
          * communicate at the
            child's level; simply
            and clearly
          * provide ample opportun-
            ity for the child to
            ask questions
          * make sure you answer the
            child's questions and
            not your own
          * try to estblish feelings
            of security and
            stability
          * provide extra warmth and
            intimacy
          Grief
          Page #543

Identify four ways of helping a child cope with death.
1. _____
2. _____
3. _____
4. _____

21/34
* don't expect too much of yourself
* don't try to deny your feelings
* let others help you
* share your feelings with others
* don't feel you must be strong, brave, or silent
* face each day as it comes
* give yourself time to heal
Grief
Page #543

Your close friend has just lost a family member to cancer. What are four things you could say to him/her that would help your friend work through their grief?
1. _____
2. _____
3. _____
4. _____

21/35
* contact several funeral directors after the death certificate has been signed
* obtain cost estimates
* ask about the funeral home's flat fee for services
* find out if the deceased had insurance that will help pay for funeral expenses
Practicalities
Page #545

Identify three tips for handling funeral arrangements.
1. _____
2. _____
3. _____

21/36
* identify a family friend or family member as executor
* list what things you own, and who you want to have them
* select a guardian for your children
* specify any funeral arrangements
Preparation
Page #548

If you draw up your own will, what are the four basic elements it should contain?
1. _____
2. _____
3. _____
4. _____

Essay

21/37   How would you characterize our society's attitude toward death? Is it basically healthy? What are some of the ways in which our culture helps us to face the inevitability of death? What about ways in which our culture distorts or denies this reality? Can you identify a culture that you think has a healthier approach to dying? If so, what is it?

21/38   Most people would like to be remembered for something after they are dead. What would you like most to be remembered for? Take a few minutes to write an epitaph for yourself. How do you feel about your legacy? Take another few minutes to select a time when you think you will die (don't worry about whether or not it's really going to be accurate). How did this exercise make you feel? Do you agree with the assertion that some sensitivity to our mortality actually enhances our appreciation of life here and now? If so, why? If not, why not?

21/39   Reflect for a moment about someone close to you who has died, or perhaps a friend who has lost a family member. Were the stages described by Kubler-Ross actually present before death? If so, how did they manifest themselves? If not, how would you describe the process of anticipating death based on your experience or observations?

21/40   There are many people who have not written a will, despite the obvious need to do so. Why do so many people avoid writing a will? If you have written a will, describe what motivated you to do it. If you haven't what are your reasons for putting it off? Are they legitimate, or just rationalizations?